Introducing nursing ethics: Themes in theory and practice

Introducing nursing ethics: Themes in theory and practice

Edited by
Stephen Holland

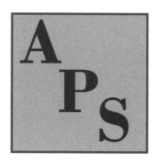

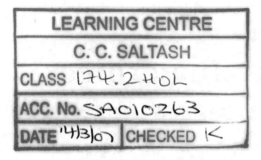
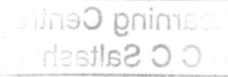
APS Publishing
The Old School, Tollard Royal, Salisbury, Wiltshire, SP5 5PW
www.apspublishing.co.uk

British Library Cataloguing in Publication Data
A catalogue record for this book is available from the British
Library

Printed in the United Kingdom by HSW Print, Clydach Vale,
Tonypandy, Wales

Contents

Contributors

H Cahill; MA, BSc(Hons), RN, RMN,CertEd: Heather is senior lecturer in the Department of Health Sciences. Special interests include consent, use and abuse of medical technology, and enhancing ethical decision-making in practice.

C Chaloner; MSc; RN; PgDip Ed: Chris is a senior lecturer in health care ethics and has over 20 years' experience as a health professional/academic. He is based in the School of Health & Social Care at the University of Greenwich where he is responsible for teaching health care ethics across a range of programmes.

C Clarke; BHSc(Hons); MA in Health Care Ethics (University of Leeds); PGCE; RN: Clare Clarke has been a Lecturer in Health Sciences, Department of Health Sciences, University of York since 1996. Special interests include ethical issues related to the end of life (treatment limiting decision) and resource allocation (micro allocation of scarce resources, age-based rationing, futile treatment).

Karen Fritz, RN, BSc, PGCE, MSc: Karen is a Lecturer in the Department of Health Sciences at the University of York, where she teaches on nursing programmes. Her background includes nurse education in her own country, the USA, followed by further studies there and in England, including her MSc at Sheffield Hallam University. She has a wide variety of experiences as a nurse in the US (from the mountains of Appalachia to near the Navajo reservations in New Mexico), in Afghanistan during civil war, in the mountains of Nepal and in the public health department of North Sulawesi, Indonesia. All of these have given her an interest in engendering in nursing students an appreciation of the richness of the multicultural experience.

Dr S M Holland; MA (Oxon); MA (London); D.Phil (Oxon); PhD (York): Stephen Holland is a lecturer at the University of York, working in the Departments of Health Sciences and Philosophy. He has been responsible for teaching Ethics to Pre-Registration Nursing Students since 1997.

A Richardson; MA; BHSc(Hons); RGN; RM; ADM Cert Ed; RNT: Aileen Richardson is currently a lecturer in Adult Nursing with the University of York. Her background is largely based in Midwifery, but her career path has enabled her to use dual qualification in UK and overseas. Interests are in Ethics derived from Midwifery Practice and through the development of reflective practice.

L Sitton-Kent; MA, BSc(Hons)RGN, BSc(Hons) DN, PGCE: Lucy Sitton-Kent is currently Intermediate Care Co-Ordinator in the East Midlands. Her main areas of interest include intermediate care, care of the older person in primary care and getting practitioners to be comfortable with research. She has worked in many areas, predominantly concerned with older people and lectured for five years at York University. She has also undertaken or been involved in several research projects.

P Warwick; MBA(Durham), PgDipHSM, PgCertAP, BA: Philip spent 17 years working in a variety of mangerial roles in the Health Service before moving into full-time education in 2000. Based in the Department of Management Studies at the University of York, he teaches on a variety of management programmes, specialising in teaching part-time graduate students. His main research has been linked to teaching problem subjects, the research being inspired by the problems he encountered trying to teach management and health policy to student nurses.

M Wolverson; RNMH.BA(Hons), Cert Ed, MSc: Mick is a lecturer in learning disabilities at the University of York. He has extensive experience extending over 21 years in the field of learning disabilities and in university education. Special interests include: ethics applied to consent, learning disabilities, and challenging behaviour.

INTRODUCTION

S Holland

This book is underpinned by two assumptions. The first assumption is that nursing is more than a job, it is a profession. The second assumption is that nursing is an especially interesting and challenging profession because it poses hard moral problems. Let us consider each of these assumptions a little further.

Many people in our society have a job and these jobs range from the menial and mundane, to the interesting and responsible. Far fewer people have a profession. It can be quite hard to distinguish between a job and a profession. On the one hand, there are some hallmarks of the professions, such as professional exams, a professional body and a code of professional practice, but on the other, it is difficult to say whether certain kinds of employment are jobs or professions. In fact, it seems to me, the most important thing about being a member of a profession is nothing to do with bodies, codes and the like, but rather with how one is perceived. Doctors, teachers and lawyers, for example, are perceived in a certain way. People recognise that they have had to work hard to get where they are, and that their work is demanding but worthwhile. Generally, they command a certain respect. Nurses receive a similar recognition because they enjoy similar kudos. When someone announces, 'I'm a nurse', it means something significant to the hearer, who immediately appreciates that the speaker has chosen a difficult, worthwhile profession that contributes something of real value to society.

The second assumption I mentioned is that nursing is a profession that is full of moral issues. In this respect, it is interesting to compare nursing with my own profession, that of university lecturer. I might occasionally encounter what could be called a moral situation. For example, a colleague might act in what seems like a less than acceptable way, or I may be unsure as to whether a student is guilty of plagiarism. In such circumstances I might wonder what I should do. But such problems arise only occasionally. For the most part I can go about the business of academia without being taxed by ethical problems. Nursing is very different. Every working day nurses encounter ethical issues and find themselves in moral situations that require sound moral judgement. Some nursing ethics issues are very dramatic, the stuff of TV dramas and films. Can we turn off the life-support machine? Who ought to get the intensive care bed? Should we covertly treat patients who have clearly withheld their consent? But just as important are the much more mundane, because much more familiar, everyday issues that are woven into the fabric of a nurse's working day. 'Who should I spend time on, this patient or that?' 'What are my moral responsibilities when I notice a colleague acting incompetently?' 'Am I allowing some prejudices to infect my nursing practice?'

Put together these two assumptions and something becomes clear. The point of nurse training is to take a trainee and help turn her or him into the best nurse they can be. This will involve learning about all sorts of things, from clinical techniques (such as giving injections safely) to acquiring a firm medical knowledge base (about anatomy, for example) to the development of social skills (for example, communication skills). But one other very important quality nurses have to acquire is that of dealing with the moral dimension of their profession. This is why courses in ethics and law are compulsory parts of nurse training. And it is the rationale for this book, which is intended to help nurses to develop their ability to recognise and cope with the moral aspects of nursing practice.

Two other points are worth making by way of introducing this book. The first is about the difference between 'morality' and 'ethics'. There are some interesting differences between these words, but these are not important in this book so 'morality' and 'ethics' will be used interchangeably.

The second point is about the relationship between ethics and the law. Usually, nursing ethics is taught alongside law for nurses, and there is an obvious connection between law and ethics. Ideally—and usually—our laws are based on ethics. For example, the reason it is illegal to download pornographic images of children from the Internet is that child pornography is immoral. But law and ethics do come apart. For one thing, ethics is broader than the law. Suppose someone decides that ethics is really very hard, so they will make things easier for themselves. They decide to act entirely in accordance with the law of the land. Would this be enough to ensure that they can live a fully ethical life? No: it would take them some way down a moral road, but they would find themselves in innumerable situations that require a moral response, which are simply not covered by our laws. And there is another way ethics and the law come apart. Although the ideal is to base laws on ethical judgements, sometimes we fail to produce ethical laws. When this happens, the issue gets debated (think about the discussions around legalising cannabis, or lowering the age of consent to homosexual sex). Sometimes the upshot of the public debate is to leave the law as it was, sometimes it is a change in the law. The point to note is that, while ethics and the law are closely connected, they are not identical and can come apart. This book focuses on ethical issues, and refers to legal matters only when they are pertinent.

One of the problems with ethics as a subject is that it can degenerate into what is sometimes called a 'clash of intuitions'. In other words, different people have different views on some moral question and their 'discussion' ends up as a slanging match as each tries to shout the other down. Ethics should be more considered than this. For this reason, some moral theories, principles and ways of arguing in ethics are introduced in *Chapter One*. These are ways of thinking about moral problems that have proved helpful when applied to nursing situations. *Chapter Two* moves on to issues that arise at the beginning of life that present the nurse with moral challenges. Abortion is very important here, so it occupies two-thirds of the chapter; other 'beginning of life' issues are then sketched. *Chapter Three* discusses 'end of life' issues. Again, there is a very dominant topic, in this case, euthanasia. Various terms relevant to the euthanasia debate are defined, and other 'end of life' issues introduced. Confidentiality and consent are two major nursing ethics themes. *Chapter Four* explains what underpins the right to confidentiality, and discusses both the nurse's obligations in this regard and the sorts of reasons that justify breaches of confidentiality. *Chapter Five* explains the right to consent, including its nature and purpose.

The next two chapters follow naturally on from this discussion of consent. Restrictive physical interventions, discussed in *Chapter Six*, are an important nursing ethics issue because the decision to physically restrain a patient has to be justified, since it might be viewed as a breach of their right to consent. And research ethics, discussed in *Chapter Seven*, revolves around the research subject's right to consent to participate in a research project.

The last three chapters of the book address broader themes that arise from the context in which nurses operate. Nursing in a society such as ours means nursing in a pluralistic society. So one feature of the current context of nursing is cultural diversity. The ethical challenges created by the increasing degree of cultural diversity are discussed in *Chapter Eight*. Another feature of the context in which nurses operate is scarcity of resources. The strain under which health care resources are placed is well known. *Chapter Nine* looks at various types of resource allocation and discusses various methods for allocating resources. Finally, the broader health care policies devised and implemented by governments and their agencies impact on the way a nurse goes about her duties. Health care policy and the ethical challenges presented by policy initiatives, are discussed in *Chapter Ten*.

1

THEORIES, PRINCIPLES, AND TYPES OF ARGUMENTS

S Holland

Introduction

Underpinning this chapter is the thought that nurses have to be adept at dealing with the moral dimension of their profession. But what does this involve? We might start to answer this by thinking about a morally incompetent agent. Suppose you ask someone why they did something dubious, and they reply, 'I dunno. I just did it.' This agent is morally incompetent because he has failed to provide any reason for what he did. Likewise, suppose someone does something dubious and justifies it by saying, 'Well, I hate blacks.' At least this agent has given us a reason for what they did. But they are still morally incompetent because their reason is a very poor one. In fact, what sounds like a reason is nothing more than a mere prejudice. Putting all this together, we arrive at an account of what a morally competent person is like. They can justify their judgements and actions by citing good reasons for them. Given this, the next question is, how do we discover good reasons for what to do? Now, this is not meant to suggest that morality is like mathematics, a series of problems with a single solution based on some formula. But it does indicate that there are some ways of thinking that, when one is considering a moral question, can be helpful. So the aim of this chapter is to introduce the reader to such helpful ways of thinking.

The chapter starts with a moral situation that can be used throughout for purposes of illustration. This is followed by three sections. The first section introduces three moral theories, namely consequentialism, deontology, and virtue theory. The second introduces the four main principles of biomedical ethics, namely autonomy, beneficence, non-maleficence, and justice. The last section introduces and illustrates some very common types of moral arguments (slippery slopes; the Golden Rule; arguing by analogy; and the doctrine of the double effect). The chapter ends with some concluding remarks about these various ways of approaching moral questions.

A moral situation

Jane and Shirley are experienced nurses on the same ward. On an especially busy evening Jane makes a mistake. In her hurry, she takes out a box of Diamorphine ampoules instead of pethidine and gives a patient 5mg of diamorphine instead of 50mg of pethidine. She doesn't notice her mistake and records the drug as being administered on the page in the drug record for pethidine. But a friend of hers, Shirley, notices the error the next day and talks to Jane about it. She tells Jane what must have happened and explains how she has 'solved' the problem. First, she has thrown away an ampoule of pethidine; second, she has written down that a patient received 5mg of diamorphine when in fact they hadn't. So now the drugs record looks accurate. But Jane wonders whether she should self-report. The patient to whom Jane had mistakenly given the diamorphine is unharmed. Shirley knows the whole story but she wouldn't say anything and no-one else could find out about it. Also, Jane knows that the culture of the hospital is such that nurses tend to keep quiet about minor errors in case they get a reputation for sloppiness. On the other hand, the hospital rules require Jane to self-report and she is proud of being an honest sort of person. But, of course, if she were to self-report, Shirley's cover-up would be exposed...

(Adapted from Benjamin and Curtis, 1992: 131–2)

Three moral theories

(a)   Consequentialism and utilitarianism

As we shall see, although it is an odd word, 'consequentialism' is one of those bits of academic jargon that is actually quite helpful. In fact, consequentialism is a moral theory that captures a line of thought that is very natural and familiar to us all. To explain, recall the moral situation Jane is in; in the scenario described Jane might well think: 'What can I do now, what courses of action are open to me? Well, I could either self-report, or keep quiet. Which should I do? Maybe I should think about what is likely to happen if I were actually to do each of these.

If I self-report then I will have blotted my copybook, and Shirley will get in real trouble. If I keep quiet, I'll feel bad—but at least Shirley is in the clear and my reputation is intact. I ought to weigh-up these likely consequences and act so as to bring about the best ones.'

In thinking in this way Jane is not being stupid or irresponsible. On the contrary, this seems to be a good way of dealing with the moral situation. And it is also clear why this approach to morality is called 'consequentialism': the moral agent—in this case, Jane—acts in order to bring about the best consequences of their actions.

For the sake of a more rigorous definition, let's say that consequentialism is the view that the morality of actions (i.e., whether they are right, wrong, permissible, etc.) is determined by their consequences. But something is missing. Nothing so far has been said about what makes one set of consequences better than its rivals. Unless we fill this in, we have the idea that one ought to do what is likely to bring about the best consequences, but are left in the dark as to what makes consequences good, so we would not know how to proceed. This is where utilitarianism comes in. Utilitarianism is an example of, or a version of, consequentialism. It says, yes, morality is determined by consequences—and, furthermore, what makes a set of consequences good (i.e., better than others, or best of all) is that they maximise 'utility' (hence, 'utilitarianism'). Now, this needs a little explaining because 'utility' is not a word we use often these days (its most common current usage is in phrases like 'utility room' and 'utility player'). So more modern words are more useful here. 'Utility' is often translated as pleasure or happiness (and, conversely, freedom from pain). But even this gives slightly the wrong impression because it sounds so hedonistic (utilitarianism is not about eating cream cakes in the bath, or whatever). So better phrases are 'well-being', 'welfare' and 'benefit'. So, utilitarianism is a version of consequentialism that says, the right action is that which is likely to bring about the best consequences, and the best consequences are those that maximise well-being or welfare or benefit.

According to utilitarianism, a moral agent—for example, Jane in the scenario above—should decide what to do on the basis of which of the actions open to her is likely to maximise well-being. This is called the 'utilitarian calculation'. Now, utilitarianism is a rather simple-sounding moral theory, but in fact it is easy to misunderstand it, so there are certain points to clarify. The first is that utilitarianism is an impartial theory. To explain, suppose someone were to ask, "I think I get it, but I don't understand whose welfare we are supposed to bother about. I mean, who counts? And of all those who we are interested in, whose well-being counts for most?" The answer is that, according to utilitarianism, the well-being of everyone affected by the action in question counts and, furthermore, counts equally. This is one of the most appealing aspects of utilitarianism (although it is also a source of criticism because it is rather unrealistic). Utilitarianism is impartial in the sense that it denies that the welfare of some individuals or types of people is more important than that of others. So, utilitarianism does not say that the right action is that which maximises well-being for myself, or white people, or straight people or the able-bodied, or whatever—it says that we should maximise well-being, full stop.

There is another important point to stress. In order to explain let me describe an imaginary scenario. Imagine you are walking quickly towards a class that is about to start.

You see a frail, elderly person having difficulty crossing a busy road because the lights are out. You decide to stop, risking missing the start of your class, in order to help them cross the road. Half-way across and without any warning, a drunken driver comes careering down the road, heading straight for you. You manage to dive out of the way, but the elderly person is hit and injured. The question is, according to utilitarianism, did you do the morally right thing in helping the elderly person cross the road? You might think that the answer is 'no' because utilitarianism says we do the right thing by maximising benefit and in this case we failed to do so. But this would be incorrect. The utilitarian distinguishes between acting so as to maximise actual benefit versus acting so as to maximise expected benefit. Utilitarianism says that we ought to act so as to maximise expected, not actual, benefit. In helping the elderly person across the road, you had every reason to expect to provide lots of benefit (a safe passage) at a small cost (being late for your class). So you did the right thing despite the fact that, in the event, your actions happened to have a bad outcome.

There is another point that can cause confusion. Most people who have heard of utilitarianism associate it with the phrase, 'the greatest good for the greatest number' (this phrase is not heard so often these days, but it used to be a well-known political slogan). This is helpful because it has kept utilitarianism in people's minds. But an important misunderstanding can arise here. To explain, let's imagine another, rather more fanciful, scenario. Imagine that you possess the last 5ml of a very unusual drug. It is unusual because, if you give 1ml of the drug to each of five people, it has the effect of curing their common colds quite quickly (they get over their runny nose and sore throats in a day rather than a week). But if you give all 5ml of the drug to one person who has a certain life-threatening condition, it has the effect of saving their life by curing the condition. The question is, according to utilitarianism, which should you do: give 1ml to the five people, or all 5ml to the one person? You might think, 'Well, if I'm supposed to do the greatest good for the greatest number, surely I should give

1ml to each of the five people—that way I help more people.' But this is not correct. The utilitarian is interested in maximising benefit itself rather than maximising the number of people who get some benefit from one's actions; i.e., it is about the greatest good, not the greatest number. So, to go back to the imaginary example, because saving a person's life is of immeasurably greater benefit than getting over a cold a bit quicker, the utilitarian would insist that the right action is to give all 5ml to the one person.

One other point is worth noting. One might well complain that it is really very unrealistic of the utilitarian to expect us to do a 'utilitarian calculation' every time we have to do something. Often, we simply do not have the time, energy or information to do this. Does this mean that we are for the most part acting immorally? No, because the utilitarian can recognise the role of what are sometimes called 'rules of thumb' in our moral lives. Take, as an example of a rule of thumb, turning up to work on time. Do we really need every day to calculate that being punctual maximises expected utility? Surely by now we have noticed that being late for work causes problems to patients, colleagues and even to ourselves, that can be avoided simply by being on time. Given this, we can act according to the rule of thumb, 'I ought to get to work on time' rather than having to keep recalculating the same moral equation and getting the same result over and over again. The point to note is that this is still utilitarianism because what makes it right to act according to such a rule of thumb is that, in our experience, doing so tends to maximise well-being.

(b) Deontology and Kant

I said that utilitarianism captures a natural and familiar line of thought. However, there is a quite different, but equally natural and familiar way of thinking in ethics. This is captured in a theory called 'deontology' (which is a horribly awkward word, but its meaning will come clear in a moment). A way of introducing deontology is by way of a complaint against the utilitarians. The deontologist might say, 'You utilitarians! I thought we were here to talk about ethics. But all you seem to be interested in is cost-benefit analysis! Of course we should be concerned about the outcome of our actions. But to me ethics is about principles. It's about doing the right thing, on principle, as a matter of duty—not second-guessing the future and doing what's expedient. If you want to be ethical, work out principles and duties and act accordingly come what may.' Given this, we can now make some sense of the strange word 'deontology', which is derived from an ancient Greek phrase that is usually translated as 'duty' or 'one must'.

There is a very clear contrast between utilitarianism and deontology here. The utilitarian says that the right action is that which maximises expected benefit. The deontologist says that the right action is that which is in accordance with one's principles and duties, irrespective of the outcome or consequences. But there is one thing to clarify at this point. What is appealing about deontology is its insistence on a role for such obviously ethical notions as principles and duty. Utilitarianism can seem rather pragmatic and expedient by comparison. This can create the impression that, of the two, deontologists are the only ones interested in ethics—that the really ethical theory is deontology. This would be a mistake. In fact, both deontology and utilitarianism are equally theories about ethics. The difference between them lies in what they say makes an action ethical. According to deontology, an action can be ethical because it is the one demanded by principles and duty, irrespective of its outcome or consequences. By contrast, according to utilitarianism, whether or not an action is ethical is determined by its anticipated consequences. There is a serious difference here, but it is not a difference between one theory (deontology) that is about morality, versus another (utilitarianism) that is not.

Let's illustrate the difference between utilitarianism and deontology, and how serious it is, by reference to a very famous dilemma in nursing. It is well known that Jehovah's Witnesses refuse to consent to blood transfusions. Suppose there is a clear-cut case: the patient is in dire need of a transfusion without which he will become very ill and die.

How would a utilitarian approach the case? They would insist that we act on the basis of the utilitarian calculation so as to maximise expected benefit. Now, of course there might well be costs incurred by undertaking the transfusion. For example, the patient might feel guilty. But let's imagine that it seems quite clear that such costs are far outweighed by the benefits of the transfusion. Suppose, for the sake of argument, that, without the transfusion, the patient will be in a very painful, life-threatening condition. Health professionals explain all this to the patient. But they get the following response. 'Yes, doctor, I understand. But what you don't understand is that I don't really care about all that. You see, I'm acting according to my religious principles. My religious duty is clear to me: steadfastly to refuse to do that which is ruled out by my faith, come what may, and that happens to include blood transfusions.' The Jehovah's Witness is being deontological, and we can easily see the contrast with the utilitarian approach taken by the health professionals.

Though it is helpful, there is a problem with this way of illustrating the difference between our two ethical theories, utilitarianism and deontology. Most of us are not Jehovah's Witnesses, and many of us do not have any equivalent, equally strongly held, religious conviction. So, to be convincing, we need an example of deontological moral thinking that could apply to us all. At this point the ideas of a philosopher, Immanuel Kant (1724–1804), are especially relevant. Kant developed a deontological approach that is based on our faculty of reason rather than any particular set of convictions (such as religion). We are all rational even if we are not all Jehovah's Witnesses or whatever. So, Kantian ethics is a deontological approach that applies to all of us. Now, there is an important point to make about the way I want to introduce Kantian ethics. Famously, Kant said that to be ethical one must treat others as ends in themselves and never as means to ends. Often, especially in books on nursing ethics, this is how Kant is presented. However, I think that although this is a very worthy dictum, it is not the best way to introduce Kant. For one thing, the utilitarian can agree with the Kantian doctrine that we should treat others as ends-in-themselves, because doing so tends to maximise benefit, so it fails to make for a sharp distinction between the two theories. Therefore, in what follows I emphasise a different (although related) feature of Kant's thinking about ethics, central to which is the notion of 'universalisability' (another bit of jargon!).

To introduce Kant's idea of universalisability, consider another imaginary scenario. Suppose a man has dashed to a bus because he just got a message to say his wife is in labour. Because it has been a particularly complicated pregnancy, it is even more important than usual that he attends the birth. The bus goes past the hospital, which is further than walking distance away. Taken unawares, the man has no other means of transport and his wallet is at home. The chance to sneak on to the bus without paying arises when the driver starts chatting to a friend out of the window. Would it be immoral of the man to sneak on and not pay? Recall how a utilitarian would analyse the situation. They would do a 'utilitarian calculation' in order to assess whether sneaking on without paying is likely to maximise well-being. They might well conclude that it would, in which case they would endorse the action. But at least some of us would hesitate. We might say, 'Well, I can see that the man is very likely to sneak on, and I'd probably do the same thing, and he has a good excuse—but, for heaven's sake, you can't call it *moral*! It's understandable, excusable, forgivable, or whatever—but it's not *morally right*.'

How can we account for our reaction here? Presumably, we are dubious about the man sneaking on the bus without paying because he is doing something that not everyone else could do. If no-one paid for their bus journeys there would be no bus service! So he is making an exception of himself. In fact, he can do what he does only because others do not. In other words, he requires that other people are paying for their journeys and keeping the bus service going so he can get a free ride. Putting this in terms of our jargon, his action is not 'universalisable': i.e., it is not the case that everyone could always do it. Therefore, according to Kant, it is immoral. So the crucial Kantian question to keep in mind is, 'is my action universalisable' which means, 'could everyone always behave like me?' Of course, very often the answer to this question is, 'yes'. For example, everyone could always be honest, kind, and considerate, and so it is morally right to act in such ways. The important things is that, sometimes, the answer is, 'no' because it is not the case that everyone could always behave as we do. When the answer is, 'no', the action in question is morally wrong.

In what sense is Kant's a deontological theory? An action that cannot be universalised remains morally wrong, whatever else might count in its favour. Specifically, it remains morally wrong even if it can be expected to bring about beneficial consequences. For example, no matter how much well-being is generated by the man sneaking on to the bus, his action remains morally wrong. And that is the hallmark of deontology: the morality of our actions can be independent of their consequences. How might Kant's approach help with Jane's predicament from the start of the chapter? Suppose, for the sake of argument, that Jane decides to keep quiet about the mistake and subsequent cover-up. So this is her action. Is it moral? It is easy to see how the utilitarian might well say that it is. But the Kantian question is, is it universalisable? Could everyone always do what Jane decides to do? Clearly, the answer is, 'no'. For one thing, Jane does not really want all nurses, all the time, to deceive their patients and lie about the drugs record. But perhaps more importantly, this could not happen. What would happen to the drugs record if everyone always did what Jane is planning to do; i.e., mis-record the administering of drugs? The drugs record would no longer exist. Of course, there might still be sheafs of paper, called 'the drugs record', containing names of drugs and quantities and so on, but they would not mean anything, not really. In order for there really to be a genuine drugs record, nurses have to be recording the administering of drugs accurately and self-reporting their mistakes. So, as with the man sneaking on to the bus without paying, Jane is making an exception of herself. She can do what she is going to do only if others do not: she can abuse the drugs record only if others are acting to maintain it.

One final point about Kant's approach to ethics is worth stressing. People often think that what Kant had in mind is a sort of science fiction story in which everyone starts behaving like you. For example, one might think that Kant is worried that if Jane indulges in deception, everyone else around her will start to do likewise, until the whole system of drug-recording unravels. But this is not Kant's idea at all. He is not making a practical point about bad behaviour 'catching on'. Rather, his point is about what kinds of actions and principles are, on reflection, universalisable. So the universalisability test takes place in the mind as one ponders whether it is in principle possible for everyone always to behave like oneself. (I should point out that there is a version of utilitarianism, namely 'rule utilitarianism'—as opposed to 'act utilitarianism'—that would rule out many of the non-universalisable actions a Kantian would rule out. But there is not time to go into the act/rule utilitarianism distinction here, or the difference between Kantian ethics and rule utilitarianism. See the 'reading list' at the end of the chapter for reading material that deals with this distinction.)

(c) Virtue theory

So far we have encountered two ways of thinking about ethics. Utilitarians say that we should approach ethics by thinking about the outcome of our actions; specifically, by asking whether they are likely to maximise benefit or welfare or well-being. Deontologists say that we should approach ethics by thinking about our duty; specifically, by asking whether our decisions and actions pass the test of universalisability. There is a third approach, called 'virtue theory'. Again, a convenient way to introduce the theory is by way of a complaint. The virtue theorist might say, "You utilitarians and deontologists, I take your points; consequences and duties are important. But what about character? Surely, being ethical is about who you are, not just what you do. It's about being a good person, a moral person—a person of good moral character."

As was the case with our first two moral theories, this seems like a perfectly natural and familiar line of thought. Consider, for example, bringing up a child (or, if you are not a parent, recall your childhood experiences of being brought up by your parents or guardians). A responsible parent has many concerns. One thing they are trying to do is to ensure that their child turns out to be an ethical person. What does this aspect of parenting entail? It seems to have relatively little to do with utilitarianism or deontology. True, parents sometimes point out the good and bad consequences of their child's actions in order to encourage or discourage certain types of behaviour. And parents sometimes say things like, "That was selfish—what if everyone decided to do that?" But, for the most part, what parents are doing is getting their child to develop a certain kind of character, or to become a certain kind of person, by ensuring that they acquire virtues. Now, this needs some elaboration because 'virtue' is another rather old-fashioned word that currently is not used much. Virtues are character traits and include things such as kindness, courage, honesty, and the like (a useful platitude here is, 'patience is a virtue').

There are a number of important and interesting points about the virtues. First, let's take an uncontentious virtue, that of being polite. How does a parent get their child to be polite? What they do not do is present their child with some kind of handbook that includes a list of situations in which, for example, it would be appropriate to say, 'thank you'. That would be ridiculous. In order to be comprehensive, the handbook would be enormous. In fact, since one could always imagine a new situation in which a polite person would say, 'thank you', it would have to be never-ending. Rather, the parent gets the child to understand what it is to be polite by getting them to 'cotton-on' to the idea in such a way that the child can then go off into the world and be sensitive to those situations in which, for example, saying 'thank you' would be appropriate. Moving to more interesting virtues, the story is the same. Take, for example, the virtue of kindness, or being considerate. A parent does not and could not write a handbook that describes all those situations that demand kindness, and what sort of kindly response would be appropriate. Rather, the parent's job is to get the child to latch on to the idea of being kind in such as way that they recognise for themselves when kindness is required and what sort of response would be a kind one. In this way, the parent is moulding the child's character.

Given this, virtue theory says that ethics is a matter of acquiring and acting in accordance with the virtues. A way of summing it up is, 'do as a virtuous person would do'. There is a very clear illustration of this theory in the scenario involving Jane and Shirley at the start of this chapter. The utilitarian might say that Jane ought to keep quiet about the whole thing because this is likely to maximise benefit. The deontologist might say that Jane ought not to keep quiet about the incident because this is not the sort of thing that everyone could always do. But the virtue theorist takes a different approach. They would pick up on features of the case, such as, 'Jane is proud of being an honest sort of person'. Honesty is a virtue. So, since in order to act in accordance with that virtue, Jane should self-report then, according to virtue theory, that is what she should do. To reiterate, this is not a matter of Jane getting out her 'honesty manual', looking up the relevant situation in the index, and following the guidelines. There is no such manual, nor could there be. Being honest is not like that. It is more a matter of understanding the concept of kindness and thereby becoming a certain kind of person, one who has honed the ability to see that the situation requires honesty, and what kind of reaction would be an appropriately honest one.

However, it might have occurred to the reader that there is a problem for virtue theory here. Honesty is a virtue, but it is not the only one. In fact, honesty is not even the only virtue relevant to Jane's situation. It was mentioned in the scenario that Shirley and Jane are friends. There are certain virtues that are very relevant to friendship. One of these is loyalty. As a friend of hers, Jane owes Shirley some loyalty. But if we focus on that virtue, as opposed to honesty, we get a different perspective on Jane's predicament. Recall that, if Jane self-reports—which would be the honest thing to do—she will get Shirley into trouble. Shirley was only trying to help her friend so it seems very harsh that she should end up being reprimanded. Surely she deserves a bit of loyalty here. For example, if Jane does self-report we can easily imagine Shirley complaining, 'Well, some friend you are!' Jane would have failed to be a good friend in the sense of abiding by one of the virtues of friendship, namely loyalty. This illustrates a major difficulty when applying virtue theory in real life. Usually in complex moral situations more than one virtue is relevant, which makes it hard to know how a virtuous person ought to act.

Despite such difficulties, virtue theory is very important, especially in nursing ethics. This is because nursing is one of those professions that really does demand character of its members. Apart from anything else, most nurses, most of the time, are extremely busy and work under great pressure. In stressful circumstances, there simply is not the opportunity to undertake the rather cerebral exercises of doing the utilitarian calculation or applying Kant's test of universalisability. Short cuts such as the utilitarian's rules of thumb can help, but nursing is such a complex business that novel moral situations are bound to arise that escape such moral short cuts. In such situations the most important thing is that the nurse involved acts on the basis of a virtuous character. That she or he is kind, considerate, courageous, courteous, and so on, is far more important than that she or he is well-versed in the niceties of moral philosophy. And virtue theory is more interesting than might at first appear. For example, consider a couple of time-honoured discussions about the virtues. First, is there one list of the 'correct' virtues that are important at all times and places, or does virtue vary with the context? Second—and relatedly—is there a connection between virtue and happiness? Some of the ancient Greeks from whom we derive virtue theory thought so. They said that a non-virtuous person could never be truly happy, and that nothing could harm a virtuous person. This might sound fanciful but surely there is something in it. We have all had the experience of suffering misfortune that does not really bother us because one's conscience is clear due to the fact that we know that we acted virtuously.

The four principles of biomedical ethics

So far this chapter has introduced the three main moral theories. Now for a change of tack. There is another set of ideas, usually referred to as 'the four principles' (sometimes, 'the four principles of biomedical ethics'). It will be worth introducing these here because the four principles are very important in nursing ethics (so they are referred to at various points in the following chapters of this book). It might seem a bit confusing to suddenly shift from the three theories to the four principles. But so long as we understand that this is not a case of 'either/or', i.e., we do not have to choose between the theories and the principles, we can enjoy the benefits of having two ways of approaching moral situations in nursing. First, here are the four principles, as originally defined in the key text (Beauchamp and Childress, 1994).

The Principle of Autonomy

This is defined as '[p]ersonal rule of the self that is free from both controlling influences by others and from personal limitations that prevent meaningful choice' (Beauchamp and Childress, 1994: 121). So, we abide by the principle of autonomy when we respect and preserve people's ability to decide for themselves; conversely, we flout this principle when we unnecessarily restrict someone's ability to be self-determined.

The Principle of Beneficence

'[A] principle of beneficence, in our usage, asserts an obligation to help others further their important or legitimate interests' (Beauchamp and Childress, 1994: 260). So 'beneficence' roughly means, 'helping others'. In healthcare, the obvious 'interest' people have is in their being in good health and free from ill-health. But there are other important interests, such as preserving their dignity and being treated with respect.

The Principle of Non-maleficence

The principle here is: 'One ought not to inflict evil or harm' (Beauchamp and Childress, 1994: 189). This makes non-maleficence seem a lot like beneficence, but it is subtly different. Beneficence is about helping people whereas non-maleficence is about not harming them. Usually in nursing ethics, the principle of non-maleficence is more stringent than that of beneficence because it is more important not to harm someone than it is to help them.

The Principle of Justice

Beauchamp and Childress (1994: 260) defined this as, 'fair, equitable, and appropriate treatment in light of what is due or owed persons'. So justice, in this sense, is about people getting what they deserve. People can deserve all kinds of things (reward, punishment, treatment, compensation, information, etc.) for all kinds of reasons (they have earned it, they are owed a duty of care, they are your friend, etc.). So we abide by the principle of justice when we give someone what they are owed.

The important point to note is that these four principles are usually at work in nursing ethics. To illustrate, recall the scenario involving Jane and Shirley. It is easy to see how each principle applies. First, consider autonomy. The key idea here is captured in Beauchamp and Childress's phrase, 'meaningful choice'. Whose autonomy, in this sense, has been compromised? One answer is, Jane's. Recall that Shirley takes it upon herself to 'correct' Jane's mistake. But did Jane want her to do this? Shirley did not even ask, she just went ahead and corrected the drugs record. Perhaps, if she had discussed it with Jane, Jane would have said, "Oh no, don't do that. I'll come clean." But she did not get that (meaningful) choice. Another answer is, 'the patient's'. Did the patient 'meaningfully choose' to take 5mg of diamorphine? No: he thought he was taking something else. So the principle of autonomy is very important in nursing because it underpins the right to consent (see *Chapter Five*). How do the rest of the four principles apply? Beneficence is about helping others, so one might say that Shirley acted according to the principle of beneficence by trying to help Jane out of a jam. Non-maleficence is about not harming others. One of the main reasons for Jane to keep quiet about the whole incident is that, if she were to self-report, this would be damaging for Shirley. And finally, justice is about people getting their due, getting what they deserve. If Jane did self-report and thereby get Shirley into trouble, Shirley might well complain that she did not get what she could expect from a friend, namely loyalty and support. She might well feel that she has a right to these in virtue of her friendship with Jane and that she has been treated unjustly by Jane.

Four types of moral arguments

The aim of this section is to introduce various types of moral arguments. It is important to note right at the start that these are very common ways in which many people argue about moral problems. They are not restricted to nursing ethics, and not even to medical ethics in general. Rather, they are the sorts of arguments that you would use in conversation with your friends in the pub. Also, note that there are other, equally familiar types of moral arguments, so the following is not an exhaustive list. Nonetheless, in my experience these four do tend to be used frequently in nursing ethics.

The Slippery Slope argument

A classic use of the slippery slope argument is in the debate about legalising cannabis. Some people argue that we should not legalise cannabis because this is at the top of a slippery slope to the increased use of hard drugs. So, think of the slippery slope argument as a kind of 'thin end of the wedge' argument. There are various points to note about this deceptively simple type of argument. For example, when people use the slippery slope argument, it is often unclear as to why they think doing one thing, which might be morally permissible in itself (e.g. legalising cannabis), will lead to something else that is obviously morally dubious (increased prevalence of hard drugs). Do they mean that the one inevitably leads to the other? If so, is this because it is logically necessary for the one to lead to the other—or is it more of a psychological claim (having got used to cannabis, we are bound to find ourselves unable to resist the temptation to go on to the next kind of drug)? So, disputes in which the slippery slope argument figures often end up in disagreements about how likely it is that the one thing will to lead to another. With these points in mind, consider how one might construct a slippery slope argument about the moral situation involving Jane and Shirley described at the start of this chapter. One response to the case is, "Well, it seems fairly innocuous of Jane to keep quiet about what has happened, but where will it end? Will she get more and more casual about recording the administration of drugs? Will she make bigger and more damaging mistakes, go to greater lengths to cover them up?" Any argument along these lines is a slippery slope argument.

The Golden Rule

The Golden Rule is a very well-known moral slogan enshrined in the Bible as, 'Do unto others as you would have them do unto you'. The idea is that we should judge how to act towards others on the basis of how we want to be treated. So if we are thinking of doing something we would not want others to do to us, we should not do it. Conversely, if we would want, or at least would consent to, others acting in a certain way towards us, then we can act in that way towards others. A very simple application of this kind of argument is, if you are thinking of stealing that fiver, ask yourself whether, if it was your fiver, you would want it to be stolen. You would not. So, you should not steal it. Again, this is a deceptively simple kind of argument. One problem with it is that it relies on people having a shared sense of what they would want to happen to them. As we well know, there is great variation between people as to what they want done to them. To take a rather frivolous example: suppose we are interested in whether certain sado-masochistic practices are morally permissible (we are interested in whether to legalise them, for example). If you ask the sado-masochist, 'Would you like that done to you?', they would say, 'Oh yes please'. But most people would not. We could rewrite the Golden Rule as, 'Do unto others as most people would have them do unto them", but this is still questionable. For example, one could imagine a society that is so racist that most people would agree to their own expulsion if it turned out that they were in fact Jewish, or whatever. Does this make expelling Jews morally right? Of course not. So, the Golden Rule is not quite as straightforward as it might seem. Nonetheless, in a context of shared norms and values, it remains a common and powerful type of argument. How might it be used in thinking about Jane's predicament? Suppose Jane is seriously thinking of self-reporting. One might say, "Hang on, put yourself in Shirley's shoes. All she did was try to help you out; now she's going to get in lots of trouble. If you were Shirley and Shirley was you, what would you want to happen?" This line of thought is an application of the Golden Rule.

Arguing by Analogy

Suppose we are puzzled as to whether some action or policy is moral. Another very common way of arguing is by analogy. The idea is to find some action or policy, the morality of which we are confident about, that is similar in relevant respects to the one in which we are interested. If we are confident that the relevantly similar action is morally right, then we can say, "since *this* action is morally permissible, so is that one". Conversely, if we are confident that the relevantly similar action is morally wrong, we can say, "since *this* action is not morally permissible, neither is that one". We can use the debate about legalising cannabis again to illustrate. Some people argue as follows: "Smoking cannabis is similar in relevant respects to drinking beer; drinking beer is morally and legally permissible, so we should let people smoke cannabis". Again, this type of argument is deceptively simple. When it is used, the discussion often turns on whether the actions or policies in question really are 'relevantly similar'. For example, referring back to the cannabis case, someone who is against legalising cannabis might insist that smoking cannabis and drinking beer are not similar in the relevant respects. They might say that there is an important difference: cannabis is a soft drug, and we know that there is slippery slope (see above) from soft to hard drugs. To this, someone else might reply, "No, cannabis and beer are similar even in this respect: there is a slippery slope from weak to strong alcohol, or from drinking socially to hard drinking". Once again, an argument by analogy might not prove conclusive. Nonetheless, it is a very common way of arguing about morality that can be very effective. How might it be used in thinking about Jane's moral problem at the start of the chapter? Jane might say to herself, "I remember a time at school when someone else got in trouble for something me and my friend had done. I came clean, even though my friend and I got told off. Afterwards I felt it was the right thing to do. That situation is a lot like the one I'm in now. So I should do what I did then—I should self-report."

The Doctrine of the Double Effect

The fourth type of argument to introduce uses what is know as the double effect. This is a slightly more difficult kind of argument, and it is important because it occurs frequently in nursing ethics. As the rather odd phrase, 'double effect' indicates, some actions have more than one effect. Specifically, they have their *intended* effect and they also have what we could call their *side-effect*. The important difference between these two effects, the intended effect and the side-effect, is that although the agent might have foreseen the side-effect of their action, they did not act so as to bring it about. They did not intend it. Rather, it is *merely* a side-effect and not the reason they acted. Let's take a simple example. Imagine (rather fancifully) that you are the driver of a train. Suddenly, at high speed, the brakes fail. You look up and see five men working on the line ahead. Suppose, for the sake of argument, that you can flick a switch that will take the train down a branch line – but, unfortunately, you can see one workman working on the branch line. You do a quick calculation and choose to flick the switch. Did you do the right thing? It might seem obvious that you did—after all, as a result of your actions significantly fewer people died in the accident. But something needs explaining here because the workman who dies was quite unthreatened by the incident until you flicked the switch. Your action brought about the death of this innocent, otherwise unthreatened workman. The doctrine of the double effect can help explain this case. Recall that the doctrine is about actions that have two effects: the intended one, and the foreseen, but unintended side-effect. In the train driver case, the intended effect of the action (flicking the switch) is to save the five workmen. The foreseen but unintended side-effect is the death of the one workman on the branch line. The doctrine is that actions (flicking the switch) that have intended good effects (saving the five workmen), but which also bring about bad consequences (the death of the one workman on the branch line), can be morally justified when those bad consequences are foreseen but unintended. To put this in everyday language, if you asked the driver, "Why did you flick the switch?" he would reply, "To save the five workmen" and not, "Because I wanted to kill that bloke on the branch line".

There are some points about the doctrine of the double effect that should be noticed. Specifically, there are four conditions that must be met if the doctrine is to be employed.

1. The doctrine is only of use when the action in question is *prima facie* (i.e. on the face of it, or, apparently) morally permissible. Going back to the train driver case, flicking the switch is not, in itself, a morally dubious action. But suppose the train driver is a

deeply irresponsible youth who has deliberately cut the brake cable simply to see what happens. He cannot then appeal to the doctrine because his action (cutting the brake cable for fun) was quite wrong in the first place.

2. The doctrine cannot be invoked if, on reflection, we have to agree that the agent's intentions really do include the bad effects of what is done. In the train driver case, this condition seems clearly to be met. For example, imagine for a moment that the brakes fail, the driver flicks the switch, but the workman on the branch line happens to be a talented amateur athlete who does a high jump out of the way of the onrushing train. Is the driver disappointed? Does he think, "Damn. Now I'll have to wait for the train to stop, go back, and shoot him"? No, of course not—he would be nothing but relieved. But other cases are not so clear-cut. In a later chapter of this book, the doctrine of the double effect is applied to cases where the doctor administers very high levels of pain killer to a patient. This has two effects: it relieves pain and hastens the patient's death. Typically, the doctor invokes the doctrine by claiming that the 'bad' effect of hastening death (although, for those who are pro-euthanasia, this is not necessarily bad) is foreseen but not intended. But is it? Or is the death of the patient really a part of the doctor's intention? We might wonder; after all, if the patient happens to linger on, the doctor might well increase the dosage.

3. There must be proportionality between the intended good, and unintended bad, effects of the action in question. What this means is that the two effects—the intended and the side-effect—must not be massively dissimilar in terms of how good and bad they are. Let's modify the train driver case again to illustrate. Suppose that the case is as above except that five workmen ahead of the onrushing train are

not working on the line, rather they are having a cup of tea by the side. Then the driver has this choice: do nothing, and the train will startle the five men who will spill their tea, or flick the switch and kill the one workman on the branch line. The driver cannot flick the switch and invoke the doctrine because the good intended effect (make sure five workman have a nice cup of tea) is obviously quite disproportionate to the unintended bad effect (death of the workman) of the action.

4. The doctrine cannot be invoked if the bad effect is the means whereby the good effect is brought about. Let's get really silly. Suppose the train driver case is just as above except there is no branch line and no switch to flick. Rather, the driver has the following choice: do nothing, and the train will career into the five workmen ahead, or grab the child who has wandered into the cabin to have look around and throw him under the wheels of the train which will grind to a halt. Can the driver invoke the doctrine to justify using the child in this way? The answer is, 'no' because the foreseen bad effect (the death of the child) is part of the means by which the intended good effect (saving the five workmen) is achieved. By contrast, in the original case the lives of the five workmen were not saved by means of the death of the one: rather, they were saved by means of changing the train's direction, the death of the one workman being a side-effect of switching track.

Keeping all these points in mind, how might the doctrine of the double effect be employed in thinking about the moral situation involving Jane and Shirley outlined at the start of this chapter? Suppose Jane self-reports. We need to ask, what is the intended effect of her action, and what is the foreseen but unintended side-effect? The intended effect is to be honest, clear her conscience, and make a public display of her commitment to responsible drug administration. The foreseen but unintended side-effect is that Shirley will get into trouble. Since the intended effect is good, the fact that there is this bad unintended side-effect does not make the action immoral.

Concluding remarks

This chapter has introduced some ways of thinking that can be helpful in arriving at good reasons for one's judgements and actions in moral situations. I want to end with some comments about what has been covered. The first thing to say is that we have only really scratched the surface in this chapter, which should be thought of as getting you started on moral thinking rather than as comprehensive. There is plenty more to say about the theories, principles and types of arguments introduced here, including different versions of, and objections to them (for example, I would urge the reader to find out about the difference between act and rule utilitarianism). And there are theories, principles and types of arguments other than the ones covered here (for example, there has not been space to introduce approaches to ethics based on the notion of rights). Some of these gaps are filled later in this book, but I would urge the reader to use the bibliography at the end of this chapter to pursue the issues raised here.

Another important thing to point out is how the various ideas introduced here relate to one another. Often, in both books and the classroom, the clashes between various theories, principles and types of arguments are emphasised. This is helpful in clarifying the differences between them, but can give a false impression, in two ways. First, it masks the fact that there are some quite clear connections between the theories, principles and types of arguments mentioned in this chapter. For example, the principles of beneficence and non-maleficence, when combined, sound a lot like utilitarianism; justice—as in the principle of justice—might be called a virtue; and a slippery slope argument is a consequentialist type of argument. Some of the ideas introduced here seem to underpin one another (a non-virtuous person would not even be interested in utilitarianism, for example). Second, it can give the impression that theories, principles and types of arguments are always at loggerheads. Certainly, it is true that they can pull in different directions, especially in those very difficult moral cases that are called moral dilemmas. For example, we saw how the utilitarian might urge Jane to keep quiet about the incident described at the start of the chapter whereas the Kantian might say that this would be immoral, while the virtue theorist might be pulled both ways depending on which virtue they stress. But this dissonance should not be exaggerated. In clear moral cases, all the theories and principles can pull us in the same direction towards the same judgement and where they do continue to clash, it is often possible to see that one or other of the approaches described here is more important to the case in question than the others.

Finally, it is very important to reiterate that the point of theories, principles and types of arguments is not to develop a method that can be relied on to churn out the correct answer to a moral conundrum. It is not like an algorithm that can be relied on to churn out the correct solution to a mathematical problem. Often there is no correct answer to a moral problem in the sense in which there is a correct answer to a simple mathematical sum. Rather, what we have here are useful ways of thinking about moral problems that can help us to arrive at more reasonable moral judgements. So none of these theories or principles is better or more important than the others; whichever happen to be relevant to our moral situation can and should be employed to help us to arrive at sound moral judgements.

An exercise

Consider how the three moral theories, four principles of biomedical ethics, and four types of moral arguments covered in this chapter might help elucidate the following scenario:

A married man comes to see his GP. Having previously been to the Special Clinic, he knows he's contracted non-gonococcal urethritis. He is worried he may have passed the disease to his wife, but he doesn't want her to know he has the disease or how he caught it. So he's told the venereologist that he will ask his wife to see their GP rather than visit the Special Clinic. He explains this to the GP and asks him to send a card to his wife requesting that she attend for a routine examination. The doctor eventually agrees because, although unhappy about the suggestion, he is concerned that, if the wife is infected, she should have treatment. Subsequently, the wife calls at the surgery in response to the request that she attend for a routine examination. She is found to have the disease so the doctor gives her a prescription telling her that she has a mild infection which will clear up with a course of antibiotics.

(Adapted from Rumbold, 1993: 134)

References

Beauchamp TL, Childress JF (1994) *The Principles of Biomedical Ethics*, 4th edn. Oxford University Press, Oxford

Benjamin M, Curtis J (1992) *Ethics in Nursing*, 3rd edn. Oxford University Press, New York

Rumbold G (1993) *Ethics in Nursing Practice*, 2nd edn. Bailliere Tindall, London

Further reading

On consequentialism and utilitarianism

Beauchamp TL, JFChildress (1994) *The Principles of Biomedical Ethics*. Oxford University Press, Oxford: 44–55

Goodin RE (1995) Utility and the good. In: Singer P ed. *A Companion to Ethics*. Blackwells, Oxford

Palmer M (1999) *Moral Problems in Medicine: A Practical Course Book*. Lutterworth Press, Cambridge: Chapter 4

Pettit P (1995) Consequentialism. In Singer P, ed. *A Companion to Ethics*. Blackwell, Oxford

Seedhouse D (1988) *Ethics: The Heart of Health Care*. John Wiley and Sons, Chichester: 103–108

On deontology and Kant

Beauchamp TL, Childress JF (1994) *The Principles of Biomedical Ethics*. Oxford University Press, Oxford: 56–62

O'Neill O (1995) Kantian ethics. In: Singer P, ed. *A Companion to Ethics*. Blackwell, Oxford

Palmer M (1999) *Moral Problems in Medicine: A Practical Course Book*. Lutterworth Press, Cambridge: Chapter 6

Seedhouse D (1988) *Ethics: The Heart of Health Care*. John Wiley & Sons, Chichester: 90–103

On virtue theory

Beauchamp TL, Childress JF (1994) *The Principles of Biomedical Ethics*. Oxford University Press, Oxford: 62–9

Pence G (1995) Virtue theory. In: Singer P, ed. *A Companion to Ethics*. Blackwell, Oxford

Sellman D (1997) The virtues in the moral education of nurses: Florence Nightingale revisited. *Nursing Ethics* 4(1): 3–11

On the four principles

Beauchamp TL, Childress JF (1994) *The Principles of Biomedical Ethics.* Oxford University Press, Oxford

Kuhse H, Singer P, eds (1998) *A Companion to Bioethics.* Blackwell, Oxford: Ch 7

2

ABORTION AND OTHER 'BEGINNING OF LIFE' ISSUES

H Cahill and S Holland

Introduction

The aim of this chapter is to introduce and discuss nursing ethics issues that arise at the beginning of life. Abortion is a major moral problem, so two-thirds of this chapter are devoted to the abortion debate. Some background to the debate is provided, then a way of addressing the ethics of abortion is outlined. The last third of the chapter introduces other important 'beginning of life' issues that present the nurse with moral challenges.

Background to the abortion debate

To give some indication of the prevalence of abortion, in 1999, the number of terminations of pregnancy carried out in England and Wales was 173 701. This equates to 13.6 per 1000 women aged between 14 and 49 years. According to the Office for National Statistics, almost 90% of all terminations are in the first twelve weeks of pregnancy; just one percent are after 20 weeks (although that is still close to 1700 cases). Of women who had an abortion in 1999,

- the highest rate was in the 20–24 age group
- 20% was married
- nearly 50% had at least one child already
- 10 000 travelled to England to secure a termination (mostly from Northern Ireland and the Irish Republic).

Picking up on this last point, the law in Northern Ireland is the most restrictive in Northern Europe, apart from the Republic of Ireland. So, although over 70 abortions were performed in Northern Ireland in 1999, most women seeking a termination travel to England for private treatment, paying a minimum of £450 for travel and medical costs. According to the Family Planning Association, some 40 000 women have travelled from Northern Ireland in the last 20 years for an abortion in Britain.

The law

Different countries have developed quite different legal formulae for regulating abortion. Within Europe these range from abortion on request in Sweden (within the first 18 weeks of pregnancy or after that with approval from the National Board of Health) to a near-complete ban in Ireland. The main legal regulations governing abortion provision in England are as follows. Sub-sections 58 and 59 of the Offences Against the Person Act 1861 provide a blanket ban on the provision of abortions. But the Abortion Act 1967 applies to England, Scotland and Wales and provides a defence against this where abortions are performed within certain specified guidelines. The Human Fertilisation and Embryology Act 1990 (section 37) amended the Abortion Act 1967 so that its Section 1 now reads:

1(1) Subject to the provisions of this section, a person shall not be guilty of an offence under the law relating to abortion when a pregnancy is terminated by a registered medical practitioner if two registered medical practitioners are of the opinion, formed in good faith:

1a) that the pregnancy has not exceeded its twenty-fourth week and that the continuance of the pregnancy would involve risk, greater than if the pregnancy were terminated, of injury to the physical or mental health of the pregnant woman or any existing children of her family; or

1b) that the termination is necessary to prevent grave permanent injury to the physical or mental health of the pregnant woman; or

1c) that the continuance of the pregnancy would involve risk to the life of the pregnant woman, greater than if the pregnancy were terminated; or

1d) that there is a substantial risk that if the child were born it would suffer from physical or mental abnormalities as to be seriously handicapped.

1(2) In determining whether the continuance of a pregnancy would involve such risk of injury to health as is mentioned in paragraph (a) or (b) of subsection (1) of this section, account may be taken of the pregnant woman's actual or reasonably foreseeable environment.

As Hewson (2001) points out, sub-sections 1a) and 1c) require the physician to undertake some risk analysis, whereas 1b) — which is based on necessity (as defined by the physician)—does not. Sub-section 1d) requires an assessment of severity of handicap (again, this is the responsibility of the physician). Note that the decision-making process does not rest with the woman. She initiates a request for a termination, but the decision to terminate is not hers; it is a medical decision taken by doctors on health grounds. Furthermore, this is a decision made by not one doctor, but two; a requirement described by Greenwood (2001) as 'irritating and anachronistic', who adds:

The law, which appears highly restrictive on paper, can be interpreted liberally by doctors who understand that it is detrimental to a woman's health to force her to endure a pregnancy and become a mother against her will (Greenwood 2001: ii2)

It is also important to remember that a woman's partner or spouse has no legal right either to demand or refuse a termination. If it becomes evident that a woman has not told her partner or spouse of the pregnancy, confidentiality (see

Chapter Four) must be maintained by the health professionals involved (BMA, 1993).

Since the passing of the Abortion Act the anti-abortion lobby has been campaigning for abortion to be made illegal in all circumstances. Their campaign has enjoyed relatively little support, and it does seem untenable these days to insist that all women whose pregnancy is unwanted must bear the child. For one thing, women would find ways to get abortions regardless of the law, resorting either to unsafe, illegal abortions, or travelling abroad. But, although it is extremely doubtful that all abortions will be made illegal, abortion law reform is still on the agenda. Liberal 'pro-choice' campaigners argue that the law should be amended to allow for 'abortion on request' in the first twelve weeks of pregnancy, with the permission of one doctor (as opposed to two, as required by the current law). It seems that the majority of doctors accept that abortions at this point in pregnancy should be allowed, and make it easy for women to meet the criteria demanded by the law. By contrast, the Abortion Law Reform Association (ALRA) proposes that there are no limits at all on the woman's choice. The ALRA recognise that, although the case for early termination is relatively uncontentious, later abortions are more problematic. Various reasons for this are cited, including that the foetus is by then 'human' and can feel pain, and that women who reach this stage should opt for adoption instead of abortion. In essence, the ALRA are arguing that abortion should, like any other medical procedure, be something that people who want it can access without having to 'prove' they need it.

The role of the health care professional

Fletcher and Holt (1995: 136) comment that, "were you not a student nurse, all the abortion debate would demand of you is that you settle your own stance on abortion". Why is abortion a specially pressing issue for nurses? A conscientious objection clause is built into the Abortion Act. This permits doctors and nurses to refuse to participate in or carry out terminations. Reflecting this, Section 2.5 of the

Code of Conduct (NMC 2002) states that the registered nurses:

must report to a relevant person or authority, at the earliest possible time, any conscientious objection that may be relevant to your professional practice. You must continue to provide care to the best of your ability until alternative arrangements are implemented.

Note that this clause applies not only to individuals of a particular religion or faith, but to any nurse. Importantly, nurses who choose to 'opt-out' of terminations are still obliged to provide necessary treatment and care in an emergency when the woman's life may be threatened (BMA, 1993). So nurses still have 'a duty of care to their patients and clients, who are entitled to receive safe and competent care' (NMC, 2002: Clause 1.4). And nurses must 'protect the interests and dignity of patients and clients, irrespective of gender, age, race, ability, sexuality, economic status, lifestyle, culture and religious or political beliefs' (NMC, 2002: Clause 2.2).

Contrary to popularly expressed opinion, women do not in general make a decision to seek a termination on a whim and, even if they are confident that their decision is the right one, they do often suffer regret and guilt afterwards. There is evidence that psychological problems occur in association with therapeutic abortion, with some 10% of women who undergo termination suffering marked severe or persistent psychological or psychiatric disturbances (Zolese and Blacker, 1992). Furthermore, certain groups of women are especially at risk from adverse psychological effects, including those with a past psychiatric history, younger women, and those with poor social support. It seems right to assume that the approach and attitude of nurses involved, and their ability to identify those who are particularly vulnerable, may be pivotal in determining how individual women respond to and recover from their experience of termination.

The ethics of abortion

The ethics of abortion is more than a topic in nursing ethics, it is one of the most emotive and intransigent problems faced by a society like ours, so nothing as ambitious as solving the abortion problem will be attempted here. Rather, a way of structuring the controversy over abortion will be outlined. The idea behind what follows is that there is not one 'abortion problem'. The ethics of abortion is more complicated than that. A good way to start thinking about abortion is by distinguishing the various questions that make up the abortion debate. There seem to be three main categories of questions, namely moral, institutional, and personal. Let's take each in turn.

Moral questions

The main question here is, Is it morally permissible to have an abortion? 'Pro-choicers' give the simple answer, 'yes', while 'pro-lifers' give the simple answer, 'no'. But most of us would give a more complicated answer because we would allow some kinds of abortions and disallow others. Which kinds? There are various, morally relevant distinctions to make. First, we need to distinguish circumstances in which a woman conceives. Contrast, for example, a woman who gets pregnant because she likes sex and cannot be bothered with contraception, getting pregnant during consensual sex with one's partner because the contraception fails, and a woman being made pregnant by a rapist or when being sexually abused. Some pro-lifers would say that such distinctions have no moral relevance because it is always wrong to kill a foetus, whatever the circumstances of conception. But many of us would be more liberal than this. For example, many of us would be more sympathetic to an abortion in the latter circumstances because the woman had not even chosen to have sex, never mind conceive a child. There are other, even more contentious circumstances. Suppose a couple know that they are at risk of conceiving a child with a severe genetic abnormality. Despite genetic counselling to the contrary, they go ahead and conceive a baby that turns out to have the condition. Is it permissible for them to have an abortion?

Let's restrict this discussion to cases of what could be called, 'normal conception': i.e., consensual sex resulting in conception due to contraception failure or 'mild irresponsibility' ("we only did it once..."). Within this category another major distinction of great moral relevance is between 'therapeutic' and 'social' abortions. A therapeutic abortion is undertaken on health grounds. There are further sub-divisions here. Some therapeutic abortions are undertaken because the pregnancy threatens the health of the mother. Other therapeutic abortions are undertaken because the pregnancy will result in a child that is very severely disabled. Finally, some pregnancies, if allowed to continue, would threaten to kill both the mother and the foetus. These sub-divisions are important because different moral arguments apply. Take a case of the first sub-division in which the mother's life would be threatened if the pregnancy were allowed to continue. Traditionally, terminating this kind of pregnancy is justified by invoking the doctrine of the double effect (see *Chapter One*). The good, intended effect of the intervention is to treat the woman; the bad, foreseeable, but unintended effect of the intervention is the death of the foetus. Contrast this with cases in which, if the pregnancy were allowed to continue, the resultant child would be very severely disabled. The justification for abortion here is different. It is based on what is known as 'wrongful life' claims. The idea is that some lives are less than worth living (imagine a baby born with such a severe disability that it can live only in very great pain, or with very high levels of sedation). In such cases, it might be argued that it is in the child's interest that the pregnancy from which it would result is terminated. Finally, in the case of pregnancies that threaten both the mother and child, the justification for termination is a simple consequentialist one (see *Chapter One*): no good will come of allowing such a pregnancy to continue.

What about 'social' abortions? The paradigmatic social abortion is one where a woman chooses to terminate her pregnancy for life-style or family planning reasons (i.e., raising a child is incompatible with her career, or she would rather get pregnant later). So the main characteristic of social abortions is that there is no pressing health need for the termination. 'Pressing' is important here. Recall, from above, that the law requires that abortions are performed because otherwise there is 'risk, greater than if the pregnancy were terminated, of injury to physical or mental health'. So, legally speaking, there are no social abortions—all abortions are done for health reasons. But, of course, this is naïve. In fact, many abortions are done for life-style or family planning reasons and justified by vague reference to 'injury to physical or mental health'. Are social abortions morally justified? Usually when people talk loosely about 'the abortion question', this is what they have in mind. Is it morally permissible for an apparently healthy woman to abort an apparently healthy foetus conceived during consensual sex for reasons to do with their life-style, or for family planning reasons?

One way of capturing why this is such a hard question to answer is in terms of rights. There are two relevant rights: the foetus's right to life and the woman's right to choose. On the face of it, both these rights seem important. Without thinking too hard about it, ordinarily we would say that living creatures have a right to life. Since the foetus is alive (an abortion is defined as the death of a foetus, so the foetus must be alive in the first place), it too has this right. The fact that the foetus is human only adds to our sense that it has this right. Having a right to life implies duties, obligations and responsibilities on others—notably, to protect and preserve the creature in question. Putting all this together suggests that a foetus has a right to life which entails a moral requirement on us to protect it. The other right, the woman's right to choose, also—at least on the face of it—seems important. Ordinarily, we assume that people have a right to choose what happens in and to their own bodies. This underpins the ethics of consent to medical treatment: what makes it wrong to impose a medical intervention on a competent patient is that he or she has the right to choose what happens in and to their own bodies. It is also what underpins our reaction to, for example, rape. What makes rape obviously ethically wrong is that it flouts the victim's right to choose whether or not to have sex. Since a pregnancy is also something that happens in and to her body, presumably a woman's right to choose can be extended to include pregnancy; in which case, it is morally permissible for her to choose to terminate her pregnancy.

Of course, the problem with all this is that these two perfectly defensible rights can clash. Endorse the right to life, and one ends up being conservative about abortion: abortion is morally wrong because it fails to respect the human foetus's right to life. Endorse the right to choose, and one ends up being liberal about abortion: abortion is morally permissible because it is what the woman chooses. So we have two perfectly sensible rights that quite obviously clash. What we need are some good arguments to persuade us to prioritise one or other of these rights. Consider the following, 'the conservative argument':

P1   It is wrong to kill an innocent person;

P2   A human foetus is an innocent person;

C   Therefore, it is wrong to kill a human foetus.

At first glance, this seems like a good argument. If this first impression is correct, then this part of the abortion debate is over: we should be against social abortions because of this argument. Since things cannot possibly be so simple, there must be something wrong with the conservative argument. But what? One thought is that there is a problem with the claim in P2 that the foetus is an innocent person. Is it? Now, it is very common—and convenient—to use words like, 'person', 'people', 'human being', and so on, more or less interchangeably. But, in moral philosophy, the term 'person' is used in a rather special way to distinguish a certain kind of creature, namely, creatures such as you and me, who have distinctive capacities, such as the capacities for self-awareness and rational thought. It is immediately obvious that, given this, 'person' does not, after all, mean (for example) 'human being'. Some human beings are not persons. A severely learning-disabled individual lacks characteristics, such as self-awareness and rational thought, so they are 'human non-persons' (none of this is derogatory towards such an individual, it is just a matter of applying the philosophical notion of 'person'). Another way of saying it is, they lack personhood. And perhaps some persons are not human beings. It is sometimes claimed, for example, that some of the higher primates (such as adult chimpanzees) have the characteristics of personhood, and science fiction is full of references to rational aliens, persons who are not human. Such creatures are 'non-human persons'. Now we can see what is wrong with the conservative argument. Even if P1 is true, P2 is false because a foetus—though human and innocent—is not a person.

Since the conservative argument fails, presumably we should be liberal and allow social abortions. But this would be too quick a response. The conservative has a reply. He says, "Well, of course the foetus isn't a person, in your philosophical sense. What I meant to say is that the foetus will become a person. The foetus is a potential person—and it is because of the foetus's potential to become a person that P1 applies to it." Given this, we can rewrite the conservative argument as follows:

P1   It is wrong to kill an innocent person;

P2   A potential person has the moral status of a person;

P3   The human foetus is a potential person;

C   Therefore, it is wrong to kill a human foetus.

Now, one thing to say about this version of the conservative argument is that the idea of the foetus being a potential person is quite a strong one. One way of explaining 'potentiality' as it is used here, is as follows. Imagine some parents who hold their new-born baby for the first time. They think, "If I can just feed this thing and keep it warm and safe, it'll grow and develop." In other words, they experience an overwhelming urge to protect and nourish their child in order to allow it to fulfil its natural, in-built tendency to develop. Develop into what? They might not put it in these terms, but what the parents mean is, develop into a person—a normal, healthy adult with characteristics of personhood, such as rationality and self-awareness. But now imagine for a moment that the pregnancy in question lasted another day—that their baby is born tomorrow rather than today. So, at the present, today, their 'baby' is still a foetus in the womb. What about its 'natural, in-built tendency'? Is it any less? Surely not. The fact that the individual happens to be located in the womb makes no difference to its potential. It still has that 'natural, in-built tendency' towards personhood. And we can extrapolate from this. It had this potential the day before yesterday. It had it last week. It had it two weeks ago. Presumably, it had it sixteen weeks ago, when it was a 24-week-old foetus.

With this line of thought in place, it seems that the revamped conservative argument is correct. But, once again, the liberal has a reply. Dwell, for a moment, on P2. P2 says two things. First, it says that a potential person has moral status. Second, it says that the moral status of a potential person is equal to that of a person. But, says the liberal, we might agree with the first of these and not the second. In other words, we might say that a potential person has some moral status and so it has some rights (or rights to some extent), but it does not have the same moral status as actual persons. It has fewer and lesser rights than does an actual person. The most important actual person in cases of abortion is the pregnant woman. So, following through the liberal response, the moral status and rights of the pregnant woman, who has achieved personhood, count for more than those of a merely potential person. Specifically, if the woman wants to terminate the pregnancy, her right to do so outweighs the foetus's right to life and protection.

This is by no means the end of the matter. This debate can go on and on—indeed, it has done so. But at least the main moves in the argument have been introduced. And to reiterate, the most important point to get across is that there are different issues under the one umbrella term, 'the abortion problem', so it is important to distinguish them when considering this 'problem'.

Institutional questions

What we call 'institutional questions' arise only if one thinks that at least some kinds of abortion are morally permissible. There are two main institutional questions. First, should (some kinds of) abortions be legally permissible? Some people argue that, even if we can, morally speaking, justify some kinds of abortions, we should not make legal provision for abortions. Take a parallel. One might think that the recreational use of certain sorts of 'soft drugs' can be morally justified, but this should not be 'legalised' because of the danger of sliding down a slippery slope towards increased prevalence of hard drugs in society (see the section on 'slippery slope arguments' in *Chapter One*). The parallel in the abortion debate is this: even if certain kinds of abortions can be morally justified, it is more important to maintain the pressure on people to lead sensible sex lives and to take responsibility for their procreative decisions. Legalising abortions will result in people being increasingly incautious and this, in turn, will result in more unwanted pregnancies and a greater demand for abortion.

Whatever the merits of this argument—and of course there are problems with, and objections to, it—it is closely connected to a second institutional question. Suppose we accept that some kinds of abortions are morally permissible and, furthermore, we should legalise them. There is still a question as to whether terminations of pregnancy should be offered as part of our public health service. The financial strain under which the health service operates is well known (see *Chapter Nine*). Is it a good use of scarce health care resources to offer 'free at the point of use' terminations of pregnancy? There is a familiar answer. Assuming—as we have—that abortions are morally and legally permissible, we should carry them out in the health service because, otherwise, there will be a return to 'back-street abortions'. Better, so the argument goes, to terminate pregnancies properly and in the relatively safe environs of a hospital, than to encourage the risks associated with private terminations. Again, whatever the merits of this argument, the point to note is that there are separate questions here: should we legalise abortion, versus, should abortions be done on the NHS?

Personal questions

There is a final set of questions worth noting that arise only if some kinds of abortions are considered morally permissible. These 'personal questions' are based on the idea that different moral issues arise for the various people usually involved in terminations of pregnancies. Of course, the most important person involved is the pregnant woman. But it is worth pointing out that she is not the only one facing moral challenges. What are the rights, roles and responsibilities of the prospective father? Does he have a right to be told of the pregnancy? If so, and having been told, what is the weight of his opinion about what to do relative to the woman's? What are the moral implications for the woman if he wants, or does not want, the child? What about relevant others, such as prospective grandparents? Finally, to reiterate, the other protagonist relevant here is the health care professional treating the woman, specifically, the nurse. Unlike other members of society, the nurse is in an ambivalent position because, on the one hand, her duty of care requires that she provide whatever support her patients need, while, on the other, the opt-out clause allows her to conscientiously object to participating in terminations.

Other 'beginning of life' issues

This section introduces 'beginning of life' issues other than abortion that present the nurse with moral challenges.

Managed reproduction

The first set of issues arises out of managed reproduction. At one time, and in some places today, procreation is a mysterious and chancy affair. However, in a society such as ours, the facts about procreation are well known and widely disseminated. Relatedly, reproduction is highly managed. There is wide variation in the kind and extent of reproductive management—from a couple using the 'rhythm method' to avoid conception, to cloning 'Dolly the sheep'. One helpful distinction is between ways of assisting versus ways of preventing reproduction. Ways of assisting reproduction include gamete donation ('gamete' means sperm and eggs), in-vitro fertilisation (IVF) and surrogacy (there are variations on each of these). For all the 'success' of Dolly the sheep, human cloning has not yet been established as a way of reproducing people. Ways of preventing reproduction are now very familiar. These include abortion (see above), various methods of contraception, and sterilization procedures, such as vasectomies.

All these ways of assisting and preventing reproduction are fraught with ethical issues (see Holland, 2003: 159–66). Some of these are very interesting but quite remote from everyday nursing practice. For example, the moral status of the embryo has been the subject of a sophisticated debate, the worry being that research and therapy that sacrifice embryos are ruled out by the moral status of the embryo (including reproductive services such as IVF which, currently, create 'spare' embryos). Other moral issues raised by reproductive management have a more obvious impact on nursing. The nurse's duty of care extends to those patients and clients who are making difficult personal decisions about their reproductive capacities. This presents the nurse with some challenges. For example, the counselling role of the nurse becomes important. Imagine, for example, talking to a young girl who is unsure about whether to terminate her pregnancy. The role of the nurse in supporting the patient or client comes to the fore. How, for example, will you talk to someone whose last chance of having an IVF baby has just failed? And the importance of non-judgmental nursing increases in these kinds of situations. Consider, for example, the following scenario:

> A young girl came in to have a prostaglandin termination. I had no firm views against termination when I entered nursing, and did not request to be allowed to avoid a ward where terminations are carried out. I had witnessed several terminations before seeing this particular one. This one, however, greatly upset me. The whole moral issue of maintaining life arose for me when this girl, of about 15 or 16 years of age, was attached to the prostaglandin pump. When she eventually aborted the foetus into the bed pan I just looked at it. It was a boy, all fingers, toes, two arms, two legs, a little hair on the head. The girl didn't want to look. There was a staff nurse present who clamped the cord. But I felt very sad inside, thinking of the women on the ward on continuous bed rest, having had previous miscarriages and desperately wanting children. I found it quite hard to be civil to the girl in the morning.

(Adapted from Chadwick and Tadd, 1999: Ch 6)

Screening, testing and immunisation

One of the major benefits of medical advancement is that ill-health can be detected and prevented very early in life. This gives rise to another set of pressing issues at the beginning of life, namely screening, testing and immunisation. Roughly, the difference between screening and testing is that the former examines a whole population to try to detect a disease or abnormality, whereas the latter tries to detect a disease or abnormality in a restricted, at-risk population. For example, all pregnant women have (or can have) an ultra-sound scan to screen for foetal abnormalities; while those women who are found to have a higher likelihood of bearing a Down's Syndrome baby can be tested by, for example, amniocentesis. Mass immunisation involves inoculating apparently healthy babies and children so as to prevent the development of contagious diseases.

Again, as with managed reproduction, all these interventions have raised difficult ethical questions, some of which are relatively remote from nursing practice. What should we be screening and testing for? Some conditions are so horrible that it seems fairly obviously a good idea to screen and test for them. But others involve value judgements that can be brought into question. Why, for example, do we screen and test for Down's Syndrome? Because we want to eradicate Down's Syndrome from our society? But why—especially since it is well known that people with the syndrome apparently enjoy a good quality of life, and give pleasure to others? At present, mass immunisation is one of the most prominent of medical ethics issues. Many parents, dubious about the MMR vaccine because of reported links to autism and other conditions, refuse to let their children have it. But this is increasing the spread of previously controlled diseases. Can we force parents to allow the vaccinations? Is the right of the parent to choose greater than the need to protect the community from the effects of their choices? There are issues closer to home, ones that impact on the day-to-day working life of the nurse. Patients and clients are making some of their most difficult decisions: do we have the amniocentesis or take our chances? If the test reveals Down's Syndrome, do we abort? If our child has the MMR and becomes autistic, we could never live with ourselves; is it better to risk measles, because then it is not our fault? Nurses are people that the public, as patients and clients, turn to for advice and support in these matters. So, once again, counselling and support are important in these situations. The good nurse—both morally and professionally—recognises how deep these worries go and responds sensibly and supportively to the predicament of their patients and clients.

Exercises

Abortion

Establish the women's position with regard to current law on abortion in the UK. Which grounds of the Abortion Act are being appealed to in each case?

1. Jemma is 17 years old and seeking to terminate her pregnancy. She has used the 'morning after pill' a number of times, but was too late in this instance. She is currently at Sixth Form College, but is unsure of any possible career direction.

2. Pat is a 35-year-old married woman with four children ranging from 3 to 14 years; she has become pregnant again by accident. Having no desire for another child, she wishes to terminate the pregnancy.

3. Rita is 31 years old and a successful lawyer. She is pregnant and believes that, unless she terminates the pregnancy, she will lose the partnership which she expects to be offered in the following year.

(See end of chapter for answers.)

Access to fertility treatment

All the following women have been medically diagnosed as infertile unless otherwise stated. It is highly unlikely that resources would be available to treat all the women. Try to arrange them into a priority list, identifying the criteria used in your decisions. Should any of the applications be refused outright? If so, why?

1. Pippa Shaw (29) and Karen Rogers (34) are a gay couple who have been living together for 18 months in a house owned by Pippa. Karen works part-time as a secretary in a bank, earning £8,000 per annum and Pippa is a supermarket manager earning £19,000 per

annum. Karen intends to give up work following the birth until the child can attend a local nursery at the age of three.

2. Jill Taylor, a lively and dynamic single woman of 58, is a partner in a firm of London solicitors. Jill currently works full-time, earning around £50,000 per annum, but she intends to work only one day a week following the birth and to employ a nanny to care for the child during her working hours. In any case she is due to retire in 2 years.

3. Jane and Peter Hindmarch, a couple in their mid-thirties, married in 1991. Peter is a trainee accountant. Jane trained and worked as a nanny for five years until she lost her job due to drunkenness in 1992 (she has been 'on the wagon' since then). She also has two criminal convictions for prostitution and one for possession of marijuana, all dating from the early 1980s, a period of her life which she says is now behind her. Jane hopes to find another job when the child reaches school age.

4. Marie Shaw is a nurse in her late 20s. Marie's husband Mike was recently killed in a car accident. Marie received a substantial payment from his life assurance company, which will enable her to buy her small house outright. The clinic had previously accepted the Shaws for treatment and currently holds some of Mike's sperm in storage. Marie very much wants to go ahead with the treatment, notwithstanding Mike's death, as this is what he would have wanted. She is confident that both sets of potential grandparents, who live nearby, will help raise the child. Mike had provided written consent for his sperm to be used in these circumstances.

5. Eric (30) and Judy (32) Jones are both teachers. Judy is not infertile but is HIV+. Eric and Judy have sought

help, as they understand there is less chance of the child being infected if it is conceived in vitro using a donor egg. However, they have indicated that, if necessary, they will attempt to conceive naturally.

Concluding remarks

A woman's decision to have a termination of pregnancy is one with which you may or may not agree. This chapter has not been designed to try and persuade you to change your mind, but rather to enable you to organise and examine your thoughts. We have looked at the abortion dilemma from an academic standpoint, but every day hundreds of women have to face the 'real' dilemma of whether or not to seek a termination. The emotional aspect of the debate can sometimes mask the very real implications that an unplanned or unwanted pregnancy has for women. Ultimately, although as we have seen, it is not really her decision to make, whether or not you agree with or accept a woman's decision is not what is important in the practice setting. What is important is that you learn to tolerate decisions that are at odds with your values and beliefs. This is what being non-judgmental really means.

References

BMA (1993) *Medical Ethics Today: Its Practice and Philosophy.* British Medical Association, London

Chadwick R, Tadd W (1999) *Ethics and Nursing Practice.* Bailliere Tindall, London

Fletcher N, Holt J (1995) *Ethics, Law and Nursing.* Manchester University Press, Manchester

Greenwood J (2001) The new ethics of abortion. *J Medical Ethics* **27**(supp II): ii2–ii4

Hewson B (2001) Reproductive autonomy and the ethics of abortion. *J Medical Ethics* **27**(suppl II): ii10–ii14

Holland S (2003) *Bioethics: A Philosophical Introduction.* Polity, Cambridge

NMC (2002) *Code of Professional Conduct*. Nursing and Midwifery Council, London

Zolese G, Blacker CV (1992) The psychological complications of therapeutic abortion. *Br J Psychiatry* **160**: 742–49

Further Reading

Cahill H (1999) An Orwellian scenario: court ordered caesarean section and women's autonomy. *Nursing Ethics* **6**(6): 492–503

Chervanak F, McCullough LB (1996) The foetus as a patient: an essential concept for maternal-foetal medicine. *J Maternal Foetal Med* **5**(3): 115–19

Dworkin R (1994) *Life's Dominion: An argument about Abortion and Euthanasia*. Harper Collins, London: Ch1–3, esp. Ch 2

Gillon R (2001) Is there a new ethics of abortion? *J Medical Ethics* **27**(supp II): ii5–ii9

Glover J (1977) *Causing Death and Saving Lives*. Penguin, Harmondsworth: Ch 9–12, esp. Ch 9

Harris J (1985) *The Value of Life: An Introduction to Medical Ethics*. Routledge, London: Ch 1; Ch 8

Singer P (1994) *Rethinking Life and Death: The Collapse of our Traditional Ethics*. OUP, Oxford: Ch 5

Answers to Exercise

All three women could lawfully terminate their pregnancies under Section 1a).

3

ETHICS AND
THE END OF LIFE

C Clarke

Introduction

Technology creates an imperative 'if we can do it, we will do it'. Ethics asks 'we can do it, but should we do it?'

(Singer 1994)

The main aim of this chapter is to identify and discuss some of the key ethical issues related to health care decisions at the end of life. It is hoped that by the end of the chapter you will have gained some insight into the difficulties and dilemmas these increasingly complex decisions pose for the health care practitioner, individuals, and society as a whole. English law in relation to end of life decisions offers little by way of certainty or logic despite the numerous 'landmark' cases that continue to generate great controversy and debate, some of which are presented in this chapter (Harris 1995).

Advances in medical technology and science and an increasingly older population have forced us to think about issues that we previously had no need to face. The development of resuscitation techniques, including closed cardiac massage, defibrillator and ventilation techniques within intensive care units in the early 1960s made it possible to postpone inevitable death (Goulden, 1994). It became almost impossible to die in hospital without active resuscitation or a mandatory period of ventilation within a highly technical and costly intensive care unit. Such courses of action resulted in treatments being initiated which brought only limited benefit and sometimes created huge burdens for the patient and his/her family. The patient's right to be self- determined and involved in decisions regarding treatment options have also been accepted, and the right of a competent adult to refuse health care treatment, including life- sustaining treatment, has gained considerable legal and moral support. However, problems arise when assessing the 'best interests' of individuals who are incompetent, because they are permanently or temporarily unable to express their wishes about treatment options. Furthermore, increased expectations about what health care treatment can and should offer has resulted in a reversal of the 'right to die' argument, with individuals and their family sometimes demanding treatment deemed futile by the health care team (Angell, 1991). The costs, both financial and human, and the inappropriateness of these courses of action have, in part, been recognised and decisions regarding withholding or withdrawing active resuscitation are being developed: but these guidelines still require interpretation and application to individual circumstances.

Key issues

- The distinction between withholding and withdrawing treatment and how treatment-limiting decisions are made in clinical practice
- The case for and against legal changes regarding euthanasia and assisted suicide
- Sanctity of life versus the right to personal autonomy
- Killing versus letting die
- The role of advance directives and proxy decision makers
- Applying the doctrine of the double effect
- The distinction between ordinary and extraordinary means of treatment.

Learning outcomes

- Define key terms

- Identify key ethical questions and issues
- Identify key 'landmark' cases
- Critically reflect on your own role, as part of a team in the decision-making process.

Definitions

Euthanasia

There is no one universally accepted meaning of the term, 'euthanasia' (Keown 1995). In 1994, the House of Lords' Select Committee Report on Medical Ethics defined euthanasia as: "Deliberate intervention undertaken with the express intention of ending a life to relieve intractable suffering". However, they also acknowledged that issues of life and death do not lend themselves to clear definitions and precise terminology. The following definitions might help:

Type of euthanasia	Definition
Voluntary	The patient's death is brought about at his or her own request.
Non-Voluntary	The patient does not have the capacity to understand what euthanasia means and cannot therefore form a request or withhold consent.
Involuntary	The patient is competent to consent to euthanasia, but does not do so.
Active	The death of the patient is brought about by an action.
Passive	The death of the patient is brought about by an omission to act.

The belief that there is a significant moral difference between active and passive euthanasia rests on the premise that there is a crucial moral distinction between making and letting something happen, of which the 'killing/letting die' distinction is a special case.

Acts and omissions, killing and letting die

An individual acts when he or she has an intention which brings about behaviour that matches the intention and is appropriate to fulfil it. An act sometimes involves physical movement, but not always (for example, blocking an entrance by standing still in order to warn someone not to enter). An omission sometimes involves not making a physical movement (for example, not feeding a patient), but may also consist of stopping something, such as the treatment of a terminally ill patient. Omissions are sometimes dependent on actions or activities because the term 'omission' often implies that something is expected, promised or contracted (Teichman, 1996: 79); for example, there might be an expectation that a patient should be treated. The essential difference between an act and an omission to act is that, where an agent acts, this must reflect intention. Where an individual omits to act, this may, but need not, reflect an absence of intention and it is the intention with which the agent acts that plays a central role in determining moral responsibility (Campbell and Collinson, 1988). Hence, what matters when assessing the morality of either withholding or withdrawing treatment is the intention with which the health care team acted. The acts and omissions doctrine states that: 'In certain contexts, failure to perform an act, with certain foreseen bad consequences of that failure, is morally less bad than to perform an act, which has the identical foreseen bad consequences' (Glover, 1977: 92).

According to the acts and omissions doctrine, it is generally thought to be worse to kill someone than to let him or her die, despite the fact that the foreseen result of both the act and omission are the same, i.e. the death of a person. Killing usually involves an agent performing an act which causes death; for example, the administration of a lethal injection such as potassium chloride. Previous analysis of an act has shown that intention plays a central role in describing the act. Therefore, the intention in performing an act of killing must be the death of the individual. Alternatively, letting die generally involves omitting to act or stopping doing something: for example, omitting to initiate cardiac resuscitation or stopping the administration of fluids and nutrition to a patient. Letting die by an omission to act may, but need not, reflect the absence of intention. Hence, letting a patient die by failing to initiate cardiac resuscitation may, but need not, show that the agent's intention was the death of the patient. Alternatively, intentionally starving a patient in one's care who is unable to feed him/herself may, but need not, constitute an act of intentional killing or murder.

Withholding and withdrawing treatment

As previously mentioned, advances in medical science and technology have enabled the lives of patients with apparently no possibility of recovery to be maintained and sustained by artificial means almost indefinitely. However and inevitably, circumstances arise when a decision has to be made to limit further treatment. The reasons for this decision, include: to respect the individual's right to refuse treatment, to avoid subjecting the patient to additional and fruitless pain, and to avoid wasting available health care resources by providing pointless or futile treatment. The British Medical Association has consistently stressed that it is the value of the treatment to the individual that should be judged, not the value of the life to be saved. Consider the following case:

> Tony Bland had gone to support his football team, Liverpool, who were playing at the Hillsborough Stadium on the 15th April 1989. During the tragedy that occurred on that day, Tony Bland's brain was deprived of oxygen and he became permanently and irrevocably unconscious. His condition is termed a 'persistent vegetative state', which is not a fatal condition providing feeding and other essential elements of care are maintained. His parents felt that, although their son's body remained alive in a biological sense, he had ceased to exist in any real sense. They asked the English Courts to declare that it would be lawful for

medical staff to withdraw feeding and other life-sustaining measures so he would die. The House of Lords eventually ruled unanimously that such a course of action would be lawful. The feeding tube was removed and Tony died soon afterwards.

(Harris, 1995)

The distinction between withdrawing and withholding treatment is relevant to this landmark case. Withholding treatment consists of not beginning a treatment in the first place, for example, not initiating mechanical ventilation or not prescribing antibiotics. Withdrawing treatment consists of ceasing a treatment once it has already begun; for example, withdrawing mechanical ventilation or artificial hydration and nutrition. (Note that the term 'passive euthanasia' is often used to describe the withdrawal or withholding of a treatment necessary for the continuance of the individual's life. In 1994, the House of Lords Select Committee viewed this term as misleading and spoke of withdrawing or withholding treatment or a treatment limiting decision.)

The belief that withdrawing treatment requires stronger moral justification than withholding life-sustaining treatment remains widely held by health care professionals (Gillon, 1994). Although the consequences of both withholding and withdrawing treatment may be the death of the patient, the former is often viewed as an act of lesser moral significance than withdrawing treatment once it has been initiated (Dagi, 1990). The justification for this belief appears to be that withdrawing treatment is equated with active killing and therefore the individual health care professional feels a greater degree of moral responsibility for the death of the patient. This is not a well-thought out view as, for example, withholding an antibiotic could be as life threatening as withdrawing the same drug since both could result in the death of a patient.

Consider the following example. An individual with end stage respiratory failure has reached a stage where s/he is unable to breathe without the aid of a ventilator. The health care team, in consultation with the patient, make an assessment of the benefit of initiating further invasive treatment and decide to withhold treatment on the basis that it would prove an excessive burden to the patient or be ineffective and provide no net benefit in terms of survival and increased quality of life. However, if the same individual was already receiving ventilatory support when the health care team made this assessment, withdrawing treatment would involve stopping or omitting to continue treatment. Hence, the only distinction is, in order to use the term 'withdrawal', treatment must have already been initiated.

In refraining from treating a patient by withholding or withdrawing life-sustaining treatment, the intention may not be the patient's death even if this is the inevitable consequence. Treatment may be withheld or withdrawn in order to comply with the patient's right to refuse treatment. Alternatively, the decision might be made to refrain from further treatment because any attempt to do so would be futile or the cost to society so great that others with more hope of benefiting from the resource would suffer. If such intentions are morally acceptable then so are the related omissions. Alternatively, if the intentions of the individual or health care team are morally unacceptable, the omission to initiate or continue treatment would be morally unacceptable.

The circumstances of the individual case are also significant when assessing the morality of either withholding or withdrawing treatment. Failing to initiate or ceasing to treat an individual whose death is inevitable is in certain circumstances morally permissible, whereas failing to initiate or ceasing to treat a patient who is only going to die because treatment is ceased may, but need not be, morally impermissible. For example, consider again the case of the individual with respiratory failure. If the circumstances arose in which there is only one bed left on the intensive care unit and two patients require admission for life-sustaining treatment, the health care team would have to make a choice regarding who receives the resource. Had circumstances been different and the resource available in greater supply, the health team might have been able to treat both individuals. The team's intention was not to allow one of the individuals to die, but circumstances made it impossible to initiate treatment for both patients. However, if the health care team failed to treat the second case and the resources were available and would not have been wasted and, additionally, the individual had not waived his/her claim to be treated, then the team would be both causally and morally responsible for the death of the individual.

There are two possible harmful consequences of believing that withdrawing treatment requires stronger moral justification than withholding treatment: it can lead to both over- and under-treatment and deprive individuals from receiving appropriate health care. In cases where the benefit or outcome of treatment is uncertain, treatment may be withheld to avoid having to maintain treatment if it proves ineffective or a burden to the individual. But uncertainty about outcome may only be reduced by initiating a trial period of treatment, re-evaluating, and subsequently withdrawing treatment should it prove to be an excessive burden to the patient or ineffective (Beauchamp and Childress, 1994: 198). For example, withholding ventilation from a patient in respiratory failure would result in certain death with no opportunity to reverse the decision, whereas the decision to initiate a trial period of treatment can be reversed, if it proves ineffective or burdensome to the patient. It is impossible to predict the outcome of treatment for an individual with precise accuracy and this can only ever be a judgment of probability not certainty.

The second harmful consequence of believing that withdrawing treatment requires stronger moral justification is that the health care team may feel obliged to continue treatment that is of no net benefit, or has become an excessive burden to the individual. This could lead to patients being over-treated or their life maintained indefinitely by artificial means and/or technology, despite there being no realistic hope of cure or recovery. However, it is acknowledged that the withdrawal of treatment appears to place more of a psychological burden on the health care team. For example, in the case we have just considered, the withdrawal of the ventilator would result in the death of the individual patient within minutes and might appear to have been the direct cause of death whereas, if ventilation had not been initiated, death would have been attributed to the terminal disease. A further harmful consequence is that individuals could refuse to consent to treatment in the first place for fear that once treatment is begun it could not subsequently be stopped.

Ordinary and extraordinary means of treatment

In an attempt to answer the question 'When is it permissible to decline to treat a patient', the distinction between ordinary and extraordinary means of treatment has been made. 'Ordinary treatment' means all medicines, treatments and operations which offer a reasonable hope of benefit and which can be obtained and used without excessive pain or other inconvenience. 'Extraordinary treatment' means all medicines, treatments and operations which cannot be obtained without excessive expense, pain or other inconvenience or which, if used, would not offer a reasonable hope of benefit (Gillon, 1986).

Consider again the case of Tony Bland. The decision by the House of Lords to remove Tony Bland's feeding tube continues to provoke great controversy. Some individuals and groups felt that nutrition and hydration are basic elements of care and that withdrawal amounts to deliberate killing. Other felt that Tony Bland had irretrievably lost all the functions, such as thinking and feeling, which made him an individual. The law lords themselves distinguished between 'being alive and having a life' with Lord Justice Hoffman stating that 'the stark reality is that Tony Bland is not living a life at all'. Is artificial hydration and nutrition essential care or medical treatment?

Assisted suicide

Assisted suicide occurs when a competent patient has formed a desire to end his or her own life, but requires help to perform the act, perhaps because of physical disability. Physician-assisted suicide occurs when a doctor gives the help requested. Whether euthanasia and/or assisted suicide should be legalised is one of the most complex and profound questions facing legislators, health care professionals and patients (Keown, 1995). In the United Kingdom and the United States of America, the law recognises no difference between euthanasia and other forms of killing. Intentional killing, even from benevolent motives by a fully competent adult, would have to count as murder. Health care practitioners are in no special or separate category and are subject to the law of murder if they end the life of a patient, even a dying patient. Demands for legislative reform have been made, but the experience of other countries, notably the Netherlands where euthanasia was effectively legalised in 1989 and subject to statutory reform in 2001, have provided little reassurance that changes in existing law would make such decisions less problematic (Keown, 1995).

Following Bland, the first recommendation of the House of Lords Select Committee was that there should be no change in the law. In their report, the Lords concluded that the interests of society must overrule those of the individual and they did not believe the arguments were sufficient to weaken society's strict prohibition on intentional killing, which is viewed as the cornerstone of law and social relationships. Their second conclusion was based on practical considerations:

'We do not think it possible to set secure limits on voluntary euthanasia. Some witnesses told us that to legalise voluntary euthanasia was a discrete step, which need have no other consequences. But issues of life and death do not lend themselves to clear definition and without that it would not be possible to frame adequate safeguards against non-voluntary euthanasia if voluntary euthanasia were to be legalised.'

Consider the case of Diane Pretty, aged 42, a terminally ill woman with motor neuron disease, who wanted her husband to be allowed to help her to die. She appealed to the House of Lords after failing in the High Court and Court of Appeal. The Director of Public Prosecutions refused to give an undertaking not to prosecute her husband if he helped her to take her life. Suicide is no longer a criminal offence in the UK, but aiding and abetting another's suicide carries a maximum 14-year sentence. The Law Lords' task was to 'apply the law of the land as it is now understood to be'. The Lords concluded, after Bland, that the interests of society must overrule those of the individual. This raises a difficult question. Is the right to die a personal affair or does society's responsibility to protect vulnerable citizens by preserving the strict rule against intentional killing outweigh the rights of autonomy of those wanting help to die?

Advance directives

This term is used to describe a document executed while a patient is competent concerning his or her preferences about medical treatment in the event of becoming incompetent. Advance directives are one category of anticipatory decision-making that competent people may choose to employ if there is likelihood that they will suffer loss of mental capacity. The General Medical Council and the law strongly support the general concept of patient choice and anticipatory decision-making: 'A valid advance refusal of treatment has the same legal authority as a contemporaneous refusal and legal action could be taken against a doctor who provides treatment in the face of a valid refusal' (BMA, 1999: 10:3). Therefore, an individual may refuse specific treatments and this must be respected, but an individual cannot demand treatment or that others assist one to die or act illegally. Other difficulties are also raised. Patients might fail to foresee the specific circumstances that might arise and make a confusing or contradictory statement. The BMA strongly advise that individuals seek medical advice when drafting the document. They also need to be regularly reviewed and dated and signed to indicate the documents' continued validity, for an individual's views might change from day to day.

Proxy decision-making is not legal in the United Kingdom. An individual cannot nominate another person to make decisions on his/her behalf in the event he/she becomes incompetent. In the United Kingdom, this decision is reached on the basis of the patient's best interests on balance of the benefits and burdens of treatment as weighed by the health care team and in consultation with family members. Family members can often identify the individual's previously expressed views but, as Goulden (1995) argues, a decision taken by the health care team based on the best interests of the patient is probably as valid from a moral and legal viewpoint as acting on the sole wishes of family members who might have their own agenda. Moreover, the individual might previously have felt unable to express his or her own views for fear these might conflict with other family members' views or he/she might have feared that increased dependence on carers rendered him/her a burden. This fear might influence his/her views and decision. However, the decision regarding treatment options is sometimes left to family members to make when in fact the decision is not theirs to make and sometimes when no real choice exists. To imply that a meaningful choice exists when there is in fact none reduces rather than enhances autonomous decision-making. This situation occurs because health care professionals lack understanding regarding the meaning of autonomy in health care, or to avoid taking responsibility for difficult ethical decision-making. Family members might not want or be in a position to make difficult decisions and choices regarding treatment options (Clarke, 2000).

Difficulties exist assessing the best interests of incompetent patients or determining whether they have any interests at all. In the case of Bland, the Law Lords declared that he had no interests, but then contradicted this statement by stating that feeding was not in his best interests. As Harris (1995) rightly argues, if an individual has no interests, he/she cannot have any best interests.

The doctrine of the double effect

Contrast the following two cases:

> Dr Cox was found guilty of the attempted murder of Lillian Boyes by the administration of a lethal injection of potassium chloride. Lillian Boyes had repeatedly asked Dr Cox to kill her and had been in intractable pain which Dr Cox had been unable to control. He recorded what he had done in the medical notes, which was reported by a nurse. He received a suspended sentence of one year and although reprimanded by the General Medical Council was permitted to remain a practising doctor.
>
> Dr David Moor, a GP, was charged with the murder of a retired ambulance man, aged 85, by injecting him with a lethal dose of diamorphine. The court was told that he visited the patient, who had had surgery for bowel cancer, at his daughter's home and, finding him in agony, injected him with a large dose of the drug. He was arrested and prosecuted after taking part in a debate in the media about voluntary euthanasia and was quoted as saying he had helped a number of patients to have pain-free deaths. Dr Moor was found not guilty by the jury at Newcastle Crown Court. The verdict was unanimous and reached in an hour.

The law recognises a doctrine of 'double effect': "On certain conditions you need not be responsible for those effects of your action which though foreseen are not intended" (Campbell and Collinson, 1988). So doctors may lawfully give pain-killing drugs with the intention of relieving suffering even if the result is the patient's death. However, they commit murder, if they give drugs with the intention of killing the patient. Dr Moor's intention was to relieve pain and suffering not to shorten the life of his patient. He may have foreseen that his actions in administering the drug in that dosage would shorten the life of his patient, but this was not his intention. The foreseen side-effects might be wanted or unwanted. For example, the death of a patient who is suffering may be welcomed, but desiring death does not mean that an intention has been formed. Had Dr Cox administered a drug with even some pain-relieving capacity, it is unlikely that he would have been prosecuted. Interestingly, in Bland, the Law Lords accepted that the intention of removing the feeding tube was to bring about his death, but decided this action was justified on the grounds that it was not in his interests to continue feeding and there was no duty to continue treatment if no benefit will be conferred.

Nursing issues: An exercise

Decisions at the end of life are becoming increasingly complex. In clinical practice, difficulties and dilemmas still arise regarding the extent of the health care teams duty of care to an individual and how vigorously the health care team should strive to prolong an individual's life. Decisions can also cause conflict and disagreement among the health care team. Consider the following exercise:

Mr Jones, aged 72 years, has suffered a stroke, which has left him aphasic and with a dense right-sided hemi paresis. His blood pressure has been very labile and he has had several episodes of hypertension, but otherwise his condition is relatively stable. He is fully aware of his surrounding and able to respond to his family. However, he is becoming increasingly frustrated when unable to converse and make himself understood. It is hoped that he will be transferred to a rehabilitation unit within the next week or so. During the ward round a member of the health care team raises the issue of Mr Jones resuscitation status. The Senior Registrar is asked to discuss the subject with Mr Jones' wife and two daughters who subsequently become very upset and insist that this decision is not for them to make and should be made by Mr Jones. However, some members of the health care team are reluctant to broach the subject directly with him in case the discussion results in additional distress and frustration, especially as he is unable to voice his views. Other members of the team feel that although Mr Jones' limited ability to communicate does pose difficulties, it does not necessarily mean that he is not competent and they wish to protect his right to information and involvement in the decision-making process.

Questions:

1. Are the family right in asserting that this decision is not for them to make?

2. What action could you take to ensure Mr Jones' views are represented and his right to information and to be involved in decisions regarding treatment options is protected?

3. The health care team are made aware that Mr Jones, in consultation with his doctor and solicitor has constructed a valid 'advanced directive', which clearly states that in the event of a cardiac arrest he does not want to be resuscitated. What are the advantages and disadvantages of 'advanced directives'?

References

Angell M (1991) A new kind of right to die case. *New Eng J Med* **325**: 511–12

Beauchamp TL, Childress JF (1994) *Principles of Biomedical Ethics*, 4th edn. Oxford University Press, United States of America

British Medical Association (1999) *Withholding and Withdrawing, and Prolonging Medical Treatment: Guidance for Decision-making.* BMJ, London

Campbell R, Collinson D (1988) *Ending Lives.* The Open University Press, Milton Keynes

Clarke CM (2000) Do parents or surrogates have the right to demand treatment deemed futile? An analysis of the case of Baby L. *J Adv Nurs* **32**(3): 757–63

Dagi TF (1990) Letting and making death happen: Is there really no difference? The problem of moral linkage. *J Medical Hum* **11**(2):, 81–90

Gillon R (1994) Withholding and withdrawing and prolonging treatment—moral implications of a thought experiment. *J Med Ethics* **20**: 203–204

Gillon R (1986) *Philosophical Medical Ethics.* John Wiley and Son, Chichester

Glover J (1977) *Causing Death and Saving Lives.* Penguin, Harmondsworth

Goulden P (1994) Non-treatment order, including Do Not Resuscitate (DNR). In: Gillon R, ed. *Principles of Health Care Ethics.* John Wiley and Sons, Chichester

Harris J (1995) Euthanasia and the value of life. In: Keown J, ed. *Euthanasia Examined: Ethical, Clinical and Legal Perspectives.* Cambridge University Press, Cambridge

Keown J, ed (1995) *Euthanasia Examined: Ethical, Clinical and Legal Perspectives.* Cambridge University Press. Cambridge

Singer P (1994) *Rethinking Life And Death: The Collapse of our Traditional Ethics.* Oxford University Press, Oxford

Teichman J (1996) *Social Ethics: A Student's Guide.* Blackwell Publishers, Oxford

4

CONFIDENTIALITY

C Chaloner

Introduction

Maintaining confidentiality offers benefits to the health care process both ethically and practically. In terms of ethical practice, confidentiality is a fundamental principle, i.e. health care workers have a moral obligation to respect their patients' confidences. Evidence that this has long been recognised as an aspect of good practice is found within the wording of the Hippocratic Oath: 'Whatever in connection with my professional practice or not in connection with it I may see or hear in the lives of my patients which ought not be spoken abroad, I will not divulge, reckoning that all such should be kept secret' (Eliot, 1910). In practical terms, the safeguards provided by confidentiality encourage patients to reveal personal, private information and thus aid the delivery of appropriate care and treatment. For health care workers, although an ethical duty of confidentiality is strict, there may be times when it is considered justifiable to breach a patient's confidence. This chapter considers the concept of confidentiality, its limitations and how breaches of confidentiality may sometimes be ethically justified.

Key issues

- Confidentiality is defined and justifications for protecting personal information are considered
- Ways in which confidentiality benefits the health care process are explained

- How confidentiality contributes to the relationship between health care workers and patients is examined
- How confidential information is acquired and managed is considered
- The disclosure of confidential information, either with or without a patient's consent, is explored.

Learning outcomes

- Understand the concept of confidentiality
- Be aware of the benefits of confidentiality for both health care workers and patients
- Reflect on the changing nature of health professional-patient relationships and how confidentiality contributes to the development of trust
- Consider the nature and range of information that is exchanged between patient and health care worker and how this information is managed
- Explore the limitations of confidentiality in health care practice.

Case study: Who 'needs to know' confidential information?

Jim Dixon has experienced long-term back pain that has interfered with many aspects of his day-to-day life. He has confided in his GP, whom he has known for many years, that the pain has been so severe, it has prevented him having sex with his wife throughout the past two years. The GP, wishing to provide the optimum treatment for his patient, has made a referral to the orthopaedic clinic at the local district hospital. Although Jim desperately wants to resolve his back problem, he is concerned that personal information he gave in confidence to his trusted family doctor, particularly regarding how the pain has affected his sex life, has now been disclosed to 'strangers' in the hospital. The GP assures Jim that any personal information will only be made available to other health personnel on a 'need to know' basis.

The disclosure of information on a 'need to know' basis seems a rational principle for health care practice; it implies that an attempt will be made to restrict access to patients' confidential details . However, although the GP seeks to reassure his patient, the principle is somewhat diminished by the ambiguity of the term 'need to know'. When information is disclosed between health care teams, it is unlikely that the identity of all those who 'need to know', either now or in the future, could be established. In Jim Dixon's case, for example, although it may be possible to identify a specific individual who 'needs to know', such as when Jim's GP makes a referral to a named orthopaedic specialist, the range of individuals working within the orthopaedic clinic, and the number of people beyond the clinic with whom they may eventually liaise, is such that it would be impossible for the GP to be fully aware of all those who may ultimately require access to his patient's confidential details. Therefore, responsibility for protecting Jim's confidences is now shared with the staff of the orthopaedic clinic who may subsequently disclose some of Jim's personal details to other health personnel, the disclosure also being justified, in all probability, by the 'need to know' principle.

Some people may feel that the information Jim gave his GP is not especially 'sensitive' and therefore its transfer between health care personnel is not morally problematic. However, regardless of whether or not the information has 'objective sensitivity', i.e. it is likely that most people would understand its need for protection, Jim's concern is sufficient to confirm both its sensitivity and its confidential nature

Introducing the concept of confidentiality in general

'Confidentiality is present when one person discloses information to another, whether through words or an examination, and the person to whom the information is disclosed pledges not to divulge that information to a

third party without the confider's permission. By defini-
tion, confidential information is both private and volun-
tarily imparted in confidence and trust.'

(Beauchamp and Childress, 2001: 305–6)

Beauchamp and Childress's description of confidentiality
indicates its two main features; the acquisition of information allied to some form of assurance that the information
will be protected. The maintenance of confidentiality serves
two broad defensive purposes. Firstly, it protects us from
the possibility of our personal details being used 'against
us' in some way; for example, consider why we are advised
to safeguard our bank account details or credit card 'PIN'.
Secondly, confidentiality (in theory at least) protects us
from the critical judgement of others; for example, why are
many people wary of revealing their age, salary, voting
intentions, etc?

Confidentiality is a familiar concept to most people. We
are used to 'keeping secrets', some of which we are asked to
keep ('Promise you won't to tell anyone about this . . . ') and
others that we instinctively know should not be made
public. It is generally accepted that personal information is
'private' and, in a sense, 'owned' by the individual to whom
it relates. It is further accepted that the disclosure of personal information should be undertaken at the discretion of
the individual. This reflects other generally accepted views
on how people should be allowed to manage what belongs to
them, for example, the sharing of personal property.

The application of the term 'confidential' to certain types
of information may suggest that it is of a 'special' nature—
one which can be objectively arranged under a heading of
'confidential'. There are certain types of information generally regarded as 'confidential', such as that relating to
aspects of personal or private life (health, finance etc)—
details of which are not usually made public. This type of
information possibly has some degree of 'objective sensitivity' (see above). However, the identification of what should
be regarded as 'confidential' is not always so straightforward. For example, disclosing a person's age may be of

great significance to some people and not to others. A shy, introverted person might suffer great anguish at the disclosure of information (their age for example) that, for a less 'private' person, might be of no importance.

Criteria for determining what is 'confidential' relate to how the information is perceived by those to whom it relates (see case study) and the possible consequences of its disclosure.

Confidentiality and the relationship between health care workers and their patients

Confidentiality is generally perceived to be implicit within health care; i.e. health care workers do not usually need to affirm the confidential nature of their contacts with patients. Although circumstances may arise when health care workers do need to confirm confidentiality, such as when a patient is reluctant to disclose intimate details of their personal life, maintaining confidentiality is commonly regarded as an integral aspect of professional health care practice.

If a person is obliged to disclose personal information, as may occur within a health care consultation, it is reasonable to assume that they wish that information to be protected; i.e. it is not necessary to ask, 'Would you like me to treat your details as confidential?' The logic of this assumption indicates that patients may have a justifiable claim (a right) to confidentiality:

> 'Competent patients have the right to control the use of information pertaining to themselves. They have the right to determine the time and manner in which sensitive information is revealed to family, friends and others'
>
> (Kleinman et al, 1997: 522)

The existence of a right to confidentiality imposes a moral duty upon health care workers to protect their patients' confidences. This right also reflects patients' right to autonomy with regard to decisions concerning what information will be disclosed, to whom it will be disclosed, in what circumstances and at what time. An intuitive respect for individual privacy also provides a basis for maintaining confidentiality. Starr (1999) discussed the concept of a right to privacy in health care. Health care workers, aware of the degree of exposure and breach of privacy demanded of patients, may therefore be instinctively inclined towards practice that both acknowledges privacy and protects their patients from undesirable intrusion.

Many of the factors that support respect for confidentiality have also influenced the changing dynamics that have been evident within professional/patient relationships in recent years. Patients' rights are increasingly acknowledged and this, together with a greater recognition of individual autonomy has changed what was perhaps a one-sided relationship into one that is, or should be, based on mutual respect and commonly agreed goals. Traditionally, a patient's involvement in the health care process was predetermined by established practices and attitudes (Loewy, 1994). Those responsible for providing care and treatment possessed knowledge and skills that, combined in most cases with an elevated social status, affirmed their authority over patients. Thus, in addition to the affects of disability or illness, patients were disadvantaged by an imbalance in both knowledge and power. Such an 'embedded power imbalance' (Gwyn and Elwyn, 1999) was most apparent within doctor/patient relationships. However, as health care provision has expanded from narrow, disease-based models to encompass broader psychological, social and economic problems, the concept of the health professional/patient relationship as a 'partnership' has been increasingly accepted. Patients have been described as 'co-producers of health services, whose potential for involvement in consultations depends on their personal rights, responsibilities and preferences' (Buetow, 1998: 243).

Enhancing the patient's role within decision-making has reaped rewards in terms of both collaboration and effective treatment outcomes (Elwyn *et al*, 1999). Furthermore, patients have demanded greater control over their care management and have been able to utilise a growing number of health-related information sources (Milewa *et al*, 2000) in addition to information gained via the news/entertainment media and, increasingly, the Internet. Thus, effective relationship development is now an inherent component of a health care worker's role (*Box 4.1*) and the manner in which patient-related information is dealt with is recognised as a contributory factor to this: 'The need to safeguard the confidentiality of the information that patients give to clinicians about their condition, their personal circumstances, their family and their way of life, is fundamental to the relationship between patients and health care professionals' (Department of Health, 1997: 2. 1).

Box 4.1: The duties of a doctor registered with the General Medical Council

Patients must be able to trust doctors with their lives and well being. To justify that trust, we as a profession have a duty to maintain a good standard of practice and care and to show respect for human life. In particular as a doctor you must:

- make the care of your patient your first concern

- treat every patient politely and considerately

- respect patients' dignity and privacy

- listen to patients and respect their views

- give patients information in a way they can understand

- respect the rights of patients to be fully involved in decisions about their care

- keep your professional knowledge and skills up to date

- recognise the limits of your professional competence

- be honest and trustworthy

- respect and protect confidential information

- make sure that your personal beliefs do not prejudice your patients' care

- act quickly to protect patients from risk if you have good reason to believe that you or a colleague may not be fit to practise

- avoid abusing your position as a doctor; and

- work with colleagues in the ways that best serve patients' interests.

In all these matters you must never discriminate unfairly against your patients or colleagues. And you must always be prepared to justify your actions to them (General Medical Council, 2001)

Confidentiality provides a foundation for trust in the therapeutic relationship (Kleinman *et al*, 1997: 522). In the pursuit of effective treatment, patients grant health care workers significant access to their private lives. The degree of exposure may be that which ordinarily occurs only within intimate personal relationships. The ability to engender patients' trust is therefore a crucial factor in acquiring information essential to the provision of appropriate diagnosis, treatment and advice. Trust formation can also have a wider impact on an individual's health care and can assist in reducing patients' anxiety while enhancing their sense of being cared for (Thom and Campbell, 1997). The creation of trust is an ongoing process that is closely related to the length of contact a patient has with a health care worker. Dibben *et al* (2000) describe how 'dispositional trust' (a psychological trait to be trusting) is dominant in the early stages of such a relationship, but that a more secure trust forms as the relationship develops. This indicates that trust, relationship development and the maintenance of confidentiality are dynamic factors that affect, and are affected by, the specific nature of the relationship a patient has with the health care service.

Although confidentiality is a key factor in generating trust and in promoting effective relationships, increased public awareness of the potential fallibility of health professionals has reduced the likelihood of professions as a whole (for example, medicine) being invested with the degree of trust they once experienced. Instead, health care workers must ensure that they actively work towards gaining patients' confidence.

Ethical and practical benefits of confidentiality

In order that appropriate diagnosis, advice and treatment can occur, patients are required to participate in open and honest discussions with health care workers. An assurance of confidentiality encourages patients to expose sensitive information, the 'cost' in terms of exposure being repaid by the provision of care.

Although revealing personal information is, to some extent, required of all patients, it is important to note that not all patients willingly submit to such exposure; a compulsorily detained mental health patient or some child/adolescent patients, for example, may well feel indignant about the process and may have little control over the range of sources from which information relating to themselves is acquired, but, in most instances, a patient's interest in receiving the optimum care will outweigh his/her interests in maintaining absolute privacy. In practical terms, the safeguards provided by confidentiality encourage patients to reveal personal, private information and thus aid the delivery of appropriate care and treatment.

Were it not for the protection afforded to personal information, it is possible that some people would be reluctant to seek health care assistance fearing the possible implications of disclosure. The establishment of a confidential health care service therefore enables the provision of appropriate treatment strategies, for both current and potential patients.

Confidentiality safeguards patients against extensive intrusion into their private affairs. The protection of information demonstrates respect for the discrete nature of the individual patient and provides evidence of the integrity of those with whom they entrust their 'secrets'. This assists in maintaining dignity and preserving individual autonomy at a time when a patient may perceive a lack of control. In its value to the health care process, confidentiality is perhaps of equal significance to some of the more overt contributors to effective care, such as the presence of skilled practitioners and the availability of effective treatment options. As such, society as a whole benefits from confidentiality as a fundamental tenet of the health care process.

Managing confidential information

Health care workers acquire patient-related information in a variety of ways. Information may be obtained directly from the patient or indirectly with their consent, by means of a physical examination for example, or via sources external to the health service, such as family members or social care/legal reports. Information that is freely given by a patient is generally on the understanding that a) it is needed to facilitate their care and treatment and b) it will not be disclosed for purposes other than this. Of course, in the pursuit of appropriate treatment, most patients' choices regarding who they share information with and when may be limited by the availability of services and/or individual clinicians.

Although the degree of personal exposure is usually the minimum required for therapeutic purposes, any information identifiable to an individual should be regarded as 'confidential' and in need of protection. However, any assurance of confidentiality must be limited as it is likely that some of the information a patient provides will subsequently be needed by other health personnel in pursuit of appropriate care and treatment. Therefore, although a duty to respect patients' confidentiality is strict, an offer of unconditional confidentiality cannot be made. Indeed, the idea of absolute confidentiality is unrealistic and would not serve the interests of the patient; i.e. the health care process would be severely weakened if patients' confidential details could not be shared within (and beyond) clinical teams. Maintaining complete confidentiality could even lead to serious harm occurring if, for example, a health care worker became aware of a threat to others that he/she was unable to act upon as a result of a stringent confidentiality rule.

Considering that both health care workers and, perhaps to a lesser extent, their patients are aware of the practical limitations of confidentiality, it is possible to view it as a 'beneficial myth' to which both carers and patients subscribe. It undoubtedly assists in advancing the health care process, although this is primarily via its contribution to the development of trust (see above). When offering any assurance of confidentiality, health care workers must acknowledge that their own duty of confidentiality (and its inherent limitations) also applies to health care personnel with whom they may share information. An individual health care worker cannot offer assurances on behalf of others—it may only be possible to reaffirm the general obligation of confidentiality held by all health care personnel—but they can indicate that the information a patient provides 'in confidence' will be treated with respect.

Patients usually disclose their personal details in pursuit of their own care and treatment. However, confidential information may also be used for purposes other than direct patient care and may be made accessible to individuals, departments and services within and beyond health care provision. It may be used, for example, to inform research studies, complement educational activities, or contribute to data gathering aimed at improving preventive health care strategies. Its use for such purposes may create tension, arising from the health service's need for information and patients' expectation that personal information will be protected and used solely for their own health outcomes. It has been suggested that only anonymised and, where possible, aggregated data should be used for such purposes (BMA 1999).

The increasing range of patient-identifiable information being retained within NHS databases led to the formation of a Department of Health committee that was established to review the non-clinical uses of medical records. The subsequent 'Caldicott Report' (Department of Health, 1997) identified a large number of flows of patient-identifiable information relating to a wide range of planning, operational or monitoring purposes. One of the recommendations of the Committee was that health authorities, NHS trusts, etc., should establish 'guardians' of patient-identifiable information: 'Guardians are responsible for agreeing and reviewing internal protocols governing the protection and use of patient-identifiable information by the staff of their organisation and must be satisfied that these proposals address the requirements for national guidance/policy and law' (Dimond, 1999a).

Patients will usually be required to supply demographic information (*Box 4.2*), some of which may be considered less 'private' than that revealed within a clinical consultation, but it is equally demanding of the protection afforded by confidentiality.

Box 4.2: Examples of the type of information, frequently communicated within the health care process, by which an individual's identity may be established

- Surname

- Forename

- Initials

- Address

- Postcode

- Date of birth

- Other dates (i.e. death, diagnosis)

- Sex

- National Health Service number

- National Insurance number

- Local Identifier (i.e. hospital or GP practice number)

- Ethnic group

- Occupation

(Department of Health, 1997: Appendix 7)

Confidentiality and sensitive information

Contemporary health care provision embraces a range of distinct specialisms. The wide variation in the characteristics and purpose of specialist areas suggests that there may also be differences in both the type of information each obtains and the degree of protection that the information demands. It may be claimed that some types of information are of such obvious sensitivity that a duty of confidentiality is particularly strict:

'It has been suggested that considering some pieces of information to be more confidential than others could ease dilemmas. For example, a patient's HIV status is far more sensitive than the fact that he or she has a chest infection.'

(Gulley, 1999: 51)

A view that certain types of information are particularly sensitive (and, by implication, have 'objective sensitivity') may be justified by examining the potentially negative consequences of unwelcome disclosure. For example, it could be claimed that details regarding an individual's psychiatric history are especially sensitive as their disclosure could potentially affect the individual's social status/employment or cause personal distress or embarrassment.

This view implies that confidentiality should be stricter in some areas than in others. However, the British Medical Association have stated that all personal information should be subjected to the same rules of confidentiality and have rejected the notion of certain types of data being 'particularly sensitive' as all identifiable health information forms a 'special and sensitive category of data' (BMA, 1999: 7). Examples of health areas where information obtained may be claimed to be of a particularly sensitive nature include:

Mental health care

Although more positive attitudes towards mental disorder have been evident in recent years, mental illness and its treatment remain a source of suspicion and fear for many. Being in receipt of mental health care remains stigmatising for many individuals and societies

Child health care

The law acknowledges the concept of 'the mature child' (Gillick v West Norfolk and Wisbech Area Health Authority (1986)) who understands the significance of proposed treatment and is able to give valid consent. It is possible, therefore, that information may be received from a child which health professionals, in agreement with the child, decide not to pass on to parents. However, the Children Act (1989) established that the 'welfare of the child is paramount' indicating that disclosure without consent is permissible if it is perceived to be in a child's best interests. Thus, the management of information pertaining to children demands careful professional judgement in deciding whether confidentiality is in the child's best interests (Devine, 1997).

Assisted reproductive health care

The Human Fertilisation and Embryology Act (1990) and its subsequent amendments acknowledge the confidentiality rights of people receiving assisted reproductive treatment and protect the interests of any subsequent children (Dimond, 1999b). Information obtained and retained via *in-vitro* fertilisation treatment, for example, may be of great significance and sensitivity to patients, and to subsequent offspring and those with whom they may have sexual relationships. In 2004, it was announced that, from April 2005, donors of sperm and eggs will lose their right to anonymity and that children born via the use of sperm and eggs will be able to trace their biological parents (The Guardian 21-1-04). Opposition to this change in the law was based on concerns that donations could cease if men and women thought they might subsequently be tracked down by unknown offspring. In July 2002, a woman challenged donor anonymity by referring to article eight of the European Convention on Human Rights, which guarantees respect for private and family life, including the 'right to form a personal identity' (The Guardian, 27-7-02).

Confidentiality and advances in health care practice

Issues relating to confidentiality in health care are increasingly complicated by developments in technology that increase the amount of personal information it is now possible to acquire. For example, the process of genetic testing raises ethical issues related to the nature and use of the information obtained (*Box 4.3*). Further ethical questions, relating to the access and storage of confidential information are raised by the use of electronic databases and communication systems.

Box 4.3: Confidentiality and genetic testing

Information obtained via genetic testing has implications for:

- **employment**: employers may try and use genetic screening to exclude from the workplace people who may develop genetic diseases in the future. Screening could lead to discrimination based on fear, prejudice and misunderstanding, leading to widespread genetic discrimination, with attendant social and economic costs

- **insurance**: genetic knowledge may adversely affect a person's insurance status in that discovery of a genetic predisposition for a late-onset condition may lead to insurance cover being refused or disproportionate increases in the affected person's premium

- **sexual partners and decisions regarding reproduction** (for example, a gene study may reveal non-paternity, or predisposition to a disease or a particular behavioural trait)

- **relatives**: unlike other clinical information, genetic information may have direct clinical relevance for other family members

The management of confidential information with regard to genetic testing raises a number of ethical concerns. To fail to respect the privacy of genetic information could discourage people from participating in research for the common good, or from seeking information which could help them to safeguard their own health. However, is it possible to safeguard individual privacy when information may be needed to protect another's life? In the future will it be possible to force affected individuals to disclose information obtained via genetic testing?

Disclosure of confidential information

'Seeking consent to sharing both acknowledges and dem-
onstrates respect for patient autonomy .... autonomy is
only protected where there is a meaningful choice made
by the patient, on the basis of adequate information.'

(McLean, 1997: 11)

The disclosure of confidential information within health care is an accepted feature of care provision. It would be unusual if, in the course of a health care consultation, some degree of inter-professional disclosure (or 'sharing') was not required. Even a comparatively straightforward intervention, such as the production by a GP of a 'repeat prescription' for medication that may not even require the patient and doctor to meet, would ordinarily involve at least the interaction of a doctor and his/her administrative personnel. Such disclosure is morally justified by the perceived benefits it affords both to patient and health care worker, and rarely demands the patient's explicit consent. Most patients' broad understanding of the health care process is sufficient to confirm their implied consent to the sharing of information in pursuit of appropriate care and treatment, although many may not be aware of the possible extent of such sharing.

Generally, a patient's explicit consent will be sought prior to disclosure for purposes that are not directly linked to his/her own health care. However, circumstances may arise when a patient feels unable to withhold consent to disclosure. For example, in a medical ward prior to undertaking a physical examination, a doctor asks a patient if he/she would object to the examination being observed by a group of medical students. In such circumstances, the patient may be disinclined to refuse for fear of being considered 'uncooperative' or 'difficult'. Therefore the validity of a patient's consent within power-imbalanced situations must always be questioned. Even when consent is given, the amount of disclosure that occurs is questionable. For example, students observing a qualified health professional require access to confidential information in order to gain skills and experience. But within these situations, it may be difficult to control the degree of personal information to which the student is exposed.

The central ethical question regarding confidentiality relates to the morality of non-consensual disclosure. The ethical justification for maintaining confidentiality is frequently stated in negative terms that indicate the 'wrongness' of unauthorised disclosure:

- A breach of confidentiality overrides the rights of the individual
- A breach of confidentiality disregards individual autonomy
- A breach of confidentiality might produce harmful consequences for the individual and/or others, as with the identification of what should be regarded as 'confidential' (see above), the consequences of unauthorised disclosure cannot always be accurately predicted.

Generally, the justification for non-consensual disclosure is that serious harm—either to the patient or others—is threatened. However, non-consensual disclosure of information may not always be a deliberate act; it may occur inadvertently, for example, via carelessly exposed patient records left lying open on a busy ward; or it may result from malicious activity whereby the deliberate exposure of patient-identifiable material occurs in order to harm, offend or otherwise embarrass someone. Non-consensual disclosure may even result from the increasing involvement of patients' relatives in the clinical process. It has been suggested that all consultations should be conducted on a one-to-one basis, with relatives being asked to leave while the patient and health carer talk. Even apparently trivial information can, if revealed in the presence of a third party—regardless of their relationship to the patient—cause distress:

'I once anaesthetised a patient whose husband had been unaware that she wore dentures until I asked her about them while he was sitting at her bedside. From that day to this I have never interviewed an adult patient without first asking any visitors to leave.'

(Aitken, 1997)

However, in most cases, non-consensual disclosure will be deliberately undertaken, non-maliciously to serve the interests of either a) the patient b) specific others, or c) society as a whole.

Disclosure in the interests of the patient

The interests of patients may be served when, for example, information is disclosed concerning their intention to self-harm. For example, if a patient 'confides' in a health care worker that he/she intends to kill him/herself, the usual response to such a threat is to consider the perceived best interests of the individual. This generally reflects a desire to safeguard their life, i.e. it is rare for the patient's decision to be routinely respected. Health care workers are able to ethically justify such a response as the aim is to enhance that individual's ability to make what are perceived to be more rational, self-determining and ultimately life-preserving decisions.

If a patient is unable, or lacks the capacity, to make informed decisions (for example, if he/she is brought unconscious into an A&E department or suffering from some forms of mental disorder), non-consensual disclosure may be an essential aspect of his/her care. The unconscious patient does not have the opportunity to consent to disclosure and acting in his/her 'best interests' will ethically justify therapeutic actions. With regard to the non-competent mentally disordered individual, benefits to the patient may be claimed if non-consensual disclosure leads to the implementation of appropriate care and treatment.

Disclosure in the interests of specific others

The interests of specific others may be served by non-consensual disclosure. For example, if a compulsorily detained mental health patient experiences paranoid delusions concerning his next door neighbour whom he has threatened to kill, the neighbour may be notified if the patient absconds from hospital. This raises questions regarding the scope of a health care worker's duty of care; i.e. is it solely to the individual patient or does it extend to others, such as the patient's next door neighbour?

A more common scenario in which disclosure may serve the interests of specific individuals is when potential or actual harm to a child or other vulnerable individual is suspected. The right of the individual to avoid harm may be felt to be more important than any right to confidentiality.

Disclosure in the interests of society as a whole

A conflict between health care workers' duty of confidentiality and obligations to the wider society may arise. In some circumstances, health care workers may feel it essential to reveal a patient's confidences even if the patient is unwilling to give his/her consent to such disclosure. The public interest influences confidentiality decisions with regard to issues such as:

- doctors' statutory requirement (under S.11 of the Public Health (Control of Disease) Act 1984) to report certain infectious diseases
- suspected criminal activity: it may be felt that the interests of justice override those of the individual patient. For example, information might be disclosed to the police, if there is a strong suspicion that it will assist in solving a crime or preventing an offence. However, in some situations, such as when a health care worker suspects that his/her patient has committed a 'minor' offence, it may be necessary to carefully balance the interests of the patient against those of society as a whole (see *Box 4.4*). The practitioner's ability to engage in critical moral reflection may

be crucial in determining whether or not he/she should report his/her suspicions. It may be felt that the nature of the harm perpetrated by the offender must be of a certain significance, if it is to justify the betrayal of patient confidentiality;

- concerns that the nature of an individual's health threatens injury to others. For example, notifying the Driver and Vehicle Licensing Agency about a patient with deteriorating vision who refuses to stop driving may be ethically justified, if the patient cannot be persuaded to notify them him or herself.

Box 4.4: Does breaching confidentiality serve the public interest?

Robert is an experienced community mental health nurse whose patient 'Francis', a 35-year-old man with long-standing mental health problems, has recently told him that he has been stealing from his part-time employer. Robert is unsure what is the 'right thing to do' in this situation. He is aware that Francis has only recently acquired his job after many frustrating attempts to gain employment.

Robert must consider the morally relevant aspects of the situation. For example:

- Theft, although legally 'wrong', can it ever be ethically justified?

- What has been stolen and for what purpose?

- His relationship with his patient: what is the purpose of this relationship? How is the relationship affected by what he has been told?

- How may the theft be affecting Francis's employer?

He must also consider what ethical concepts are relevant to the situation. For example:

- His ethical (and professional) duty; does he have a duty to inform someone about the theft; i.e. none of the above aspects should inform his decision-making, he should simple report the theft?

- Respect for autonomy: could Robert justify overriding Francis's autonomy by informing others of the possible theft?

- The best interests of Francis (and the best interests of Robert)

- Rights: does Francis have the right to confidentiality? Do others (e.g. Francis's employer) have a right to be told this information?

- Avoidance of harm: if Robert seeks to avoid or at least minimise harm, what is the most appropriate action for him to take? How can he define 'harm' in this instance?

By carefully considering the morally relevant aspects and key ethical concepts, it may be possible for Robert to reach an ethical conclusion. This does not have to be one that is agreed by others, but it must be one that Robert himself can ethically justify.

(Chaloner, 2003:45)

Exercise

This exercise concerns confidentiality and a health care worker's duty of care:

A GP is informed by her HIV positive patient that he (the patient) intends to continue having unprotected sex with his partner who is unaware of his diagnosis. The doctor wishes to protect the confidentiality of her patient but is aware that this may lead to harm occurring to the patient's partner.

Questions

1. Do patients have an 'absolute right to confidentiality' when they consult their GP?

2. Does a GP have the right to decide with whom he/she will share his/her patients' confidential details?

3. How can the GP morally justify informing her patient's partner of the patient's HIV status?

4. To what extent does the patient's partner's right to avoid harm influence the GP's decision-making?

5. Is the GP's duty of confidentiality solely to her patient or does it also extend to the patient's partner?

6. Could the doctor be 'morally guilty' of any harm that may result from not informing the patient's partner?

7. What are the potential consequences if it is perceived that GPs do not protect their patients' confidences?

8. What should the GP do in this case? How can she achieve a justified response to her 'moral dilemma'?

Summary

Effective health care depends upon the exchange of relevant information between patients and health care workers. Although the maintenance of confidentiality should not be regarded as an absolute concept, as information may be disclosed for many reasons, it is central to the successful provision of health care and the ethical duties of health care workers. Confidentiality encourages patients to seek out health care and participate in their own care and treatment; it acknowledges individual autonomy and rights while imposing moral obligations on health care personnel. Disclosure of confidential information ordinarily occurs with a patient's implicit or explicit consent, although non-consensual disclosure may sometimes be necessary—and ethically justified.

References

Aitken H (1997) A salutary lesson: family secrets. *Br Med J* **314**: 1718

Beauchamp T, Childress J (2001) *Principles of Biomedical Ethics*, 5th edn. Oxford University Press, Oxford

British Medical Association (1999). *Confidentiality and Disclosure of Health Information*. BMA, London

Buetow S (1998) The scope for the involvement of patients in their consultations with health professionals: rights, responsibilities and preferences of patients. *J Medical Ethics* **24**(4): 243–47

Chaloner C (2003) Ethical issues. In: Hannigan B, Coffey M, Burnard P, eds. A Handbook of community Psychiatric Nursing. Routledge, London: Ch 4

Department of Health (1997) *Report on the Review of Patient-Identifiable Information*. HMSO, London

Devine M (1997) Care and secrets. *Nurs Times* **93**(46): 30

Dibben MR, Morris SE, Lean ME (2000) Situational trust and co-operative partnerships between physicians and their patients: A theoretical explanation transferable from business practice. *QJM* **93**(1): 55–61

Dimond B (1999a) Confidentiality 8: role of the NHS trust and patient confidentiality. *Br J Nurs* **8**(17): 1176

Dimond B (1999b) Confidentiality 7: human fertilization and embryology issues. *Br J Nurs* **8**(17): 1176

Eliot CW ed (1910) *Scientific Papers: Physiology, Medicine, Surgery, Geology*. (Harvard Classics Vol. 38). P F Collier and Son Co. New York

Elwyn G, Edwards A, Gwyn R Grol R (1999). Towards a feasible model for shared decision making: focus group study with general practice registrars. *Br Med J* **319**(7212): 753–56

General Medical Council (2001) *Good Medical Practice*, 3rd edn. General Medical Council, London

Gulley S (1999) Dealing with the dilemmas of confidentiality. *Nurs Times* **95**(1): 50–51

Gwyn R, Elwyn G (1999) When is a shared decision not (quite) a shared decision? Negotiating preferences in a general practice encounter. *Soc Sci Med* **49**(4): 437–47

Loewy RS (1994) A critique of traditional relationship models. *Camb Q J Health Care Ethics* **3**(1): 27–37

Kleinman I, Balis F, Rodgers S, Singer P (1997) Bioethics for clinicians: 8. Confidentiality. *Can Medic Assoc J* **156**(4): 521–24

McLean S (1997) *Consent and The Law*. Review of the Current Provisions in the Human Fertilisation and Embryology Act 1990 for the UK Health Ministers. Glasgow University / Department of Health

Milewa T, Calnan M, Almond S, Hunter A (2000) Patient education literature and help seeking behaviour: perspectives from an evaluation in the United Kingdom. *Soc Sci Med* **51**(3): 463–75

Starr P (1999) Health and the right to privacy. *Am J Law Med* **25**: 193–201

The Guardian (21-1-04) Sperm donors to lose anonymity. *Guardian*

The Guardian (27-7-02) Hope for Sperm Donor Offspring. *Guardian*

Thom D, Campbell B (1997) Patient-Physician Trust: An exploratory study. *J Fam Pract* **44**(2): 169–76

Further reading

Dimond B (2002) *Legal Aspects of Patient Confidentiality*. British Journal of Nursing Monograph. Quay Books, Wiltshire

Although this book focuses primarily on the legal aspects of confidentiality it also discusses many of the issues addressed within this chapter. It is a short 'accessible' text that makes effective use of case scenarios to highlight relevant issues.

Cordess C, ed. (2001) *Confidentiality and Mental Health.* Jessica Kingsley Publishers, London

Each of the chapters of this book is devoted to one specific aspect of confidentiality within mental health care. A wide range of issues are explored including many that are relevant to the 'confidentiality dilemmas' faced by all health care workers.

5

CONSENT

H Cahill

Introduction

'Understanding of the key concepts of consent is vital for safe practice. All practitioners must be aware of the boundaries and implications of their duty of care to patients and understand the position of the law.'

(Cahill, 1998: 3)

Codes of practice laid down by statute clearly establish that health professionals owe a duty of care to patients, a duty that is founded in the special relationship between themselves and those for whom they care. There are a number of different ways in which this duty can be expressed, but one of the most important is the duty to ensure that consent is obtained prior to any intervention. In this chapter, we will:

- examine the ethical principles underpinning consent
- explore the nature and purposes of consent
- discuss the implications of invalid consent for professionals and patients
- explore the essential legal criteria of consent
- clarify the policy requirements of consent in practice.

The nature and purpose of consent

Consent expresses respect for autonomy in much the same way as an apology expresses regret (Dworkin, 1988); without the latter, the former is rendered meaningless. In practice, many doctors and nurses have seen consent purely in medico-legal terms, focussing on the requirement of patients to sign a form (Kessel, 1994). Kennedy (1992: 49) rightly describes health care professionals' understanding of consent as a 'triumph of myth over reality'. Too many doctors, and nurses it would seem, still believe that consent can only be valid when it is in writing and that something in writing is all that is required for consent to be valid. In fact, consent can be express (verbal or in writing) or implied and the law sees no difference in importance between them (Dimond, 1995). The validity of consent is not dependent on the form in which authorisation is given: written consent merely serves as evidence. As Worthington (2002: 377) puts it, 'the ethical validity of consent hinges not on the written word, but the nature and quality of the interaction between patient and clinician'. If the crucial standards of voluntariness, capacity and disclosure (see later in the chapter) have not been met, a signature on a form will not make consent valid. As the Department of Health has made clear, 'a signature on a form is *evidence* that the patient has given consent, but is not *proof* of valid consent' (Department of Health, 2001a). The courts will be the final arbiters of what constitutes reasonable practice.

So let us first establish that consent is much more than a signature on a form. When obtaining consent, the doctor or nurse is explicitly according respect to patients' wishes. In other words, respect for patients' autonomy assumes greater authority than an assessment of their best interests and, according to Gillon (1986), it is the principle of respect for autonomy that underpins the requirements of consent. The right to determine one's own life, already an established principle in law, was reaffirmed by the House of Lords judgement in the case of Anthony Bland: 'the principle of the sanctity of life must yield to that of the right to self-determination' (Mason and McCall Smith, 1994: 342).

Consent serves two distinct purposes (Montgomery, 2002). Firstly, it provides the legal justification for care and treatment and, secondly, it secures patients' trust and co-operation. Montgomery also points out that the securing of trust and co-operation requires more in the way of detailed information than the law associated with legal justification of treatment actually requires. In a similar vein, Downie and Calman (1994) describe consent as a legal device designed to protect individuals and their autonomy, as legal protection for professionals and, crucially, as an extension of a relationship that is based on trust. Consent therefore relates not just to participation in research or consent to treatment, but to any relationship between health care professionals and patients (Cahill and Jackson, 1997).

What constitutes a valid consent?

Consent is concerned with respecting and safeguarding patients' rights to self-determination. Therefore, it requires disclosure and sound communication skills on the part of the clinician, and, from the patient, understanding, voluntary agreement, competence and authorisation (McLean and Maher, 1993). Beauchamp and Childress (2001) outline the three groups of elements of valid consent:

(1) Threshold elements
The threshold elements are competence (i.e. the patient/ client must be able to understand and decide) and voluntariness (i.e. the decision is free from coercion—be that coercion subtle or otherwise—in other words, consent must be voluntary). Competence (sometimes referred to as capacity) is difficult both to define and standardise (Beauchamp and Childress, 2001) yet, in the context of consent, is taken to mean that patients understand in broad terms to what it is they are consenting. Importantly, competence should be presumed to be present rather than absent. As Montgomery (2002) points out, explicit evidence that an individual could not understand the proposed procedure or treatment would be required. Temporary factors, such as pain, fatigue or drugs, may erode capacity, but those health care professionals concerned must be satisfied that they are at such a level that the ability to decide is absent. In 1997, the NHS Executive sought to remind all practitioners that, while indecisiveness, panic and irrationality may be symptoms of incompetence, they do not actually define incompetence.

Remember that competence, like autonomy, is not an absolute. The focus should always be on the quality of the individual decision rather than on, often mistaken, assumptions about different patient groups.

The case of Re C in 1994, the only reported case in
common law in which the autonomy of a compulsorily-
detained patient has been upheld, concerned the capacity of
a paranoid patient to refuse amputation of his gangrenous
leg. Justice Thorpe applied a three-strand test of competence in this case, namely:

(i)   Whether or not the individual is capable of understand-
        ing and retaining information about the treatment;

(ii)   Whether or not the individual is capable of believing
        that information;

(iii)   Whether or not the individual is capable of weighing
        it in the balance to make a choice.

That patients/clients in Justice Thorpe's test appear to be
required to believe all medical advice to be considered competent is rather questionable. While doctors clearly have a
moral obligation to provide accurate information and to
clarify options, it must be recognised that medical advice is
based on evidence that is rarely infallible: 'It is an expression of best judgement, not an absolute truth' (McMillan,
1995: 114). This is an important distinction, as doctors have
been known to disagree about the character and utilisation
of different interventions and therefore any prediction of
harm will be at best uncertain.

(2) Information elements

Disclosure is a two-way requirement on both practitioner and patient/client. Acting on beneficent obligations
towards patients too often leads to paternalistic assessments of their best interests (Faulder, 1985) and this is frequently reflected in individual clinicians' assessments of
what information it is necessary to disclose. Clearly a proposed intervention can be (in the clinicians' best

judgement) either the only feasible option or the best option. Despite any beneficent intentions, to give the impression that the former is the case when in fact it is the latter is to coerce by deception. And remember, coercion invalidates consent regardless of good intention. The practitioner should therefore provide information about the nature of the proposed treatment in broad terms, why it has been prescribed, its principal benefits and risks, and the consequences of not having the treatment. The patient/client should disclose their feelings and views about their illness and its management. For example, a below-knee amputation might be the best course of action as defined by a vascular surgeon, but may be the last option in the mind of a patient/client for whom independence is crucial.

The upshot of a consultation between doctor and patient is the recommendation of a plan by the former to the latter. Understanding the plan is vital to consent. It is the duty of the person obtaining consent to assess the level of understanding and assimilation of the information disclosed and the recommended plan. Remember that there is a very real difference between being in the possession of, and really understanding, certain facts. The Department of Health (2001a) reminds all practitioners that acquiescence where the patient does not understand what the intervention entails, but still signs a form, is not consent.

(3) Consent elements

Concerning the decision made by the patient/client to accept or refuse a proposed intervention, Robinson (1995) makes the important point that the terms 'informed' and 'consent' seem to be automatically linked; it rarely seems to occur to doctors and nurses that once being so informed, a patient/client may refuse a treatment option on the basis of that information. Evidently, there is a distinct difference between accepting someone as competent and actually acceding to their decision-making. It is as if the entrenched beliefs of some doctors that they know what are patients' best interests have been translated into what Draper (1996a) has described as a faulty argument that runs as follows: 'I (the doctor) am the expert and you (the patient/client) would be foolish to ignore my advice. You are ignoring my advice, therefore you are foolish and irresponsible. Because you are foolish and irresponsible, you are not competent to make this decision. I am, therefore, wholly justified in overriding your foolhardy and irresponsible wishes'. But again remember that competence is not an absolute. Patients sometimes do reject professional advice for a variety of reasons, be they rational or otherwise, but it is important to remember that such a rejection is not evidence of incompetence. Perhaps, as Draper (1996b) suggests, patients are only given the freedom to choose those treatment options that would be chosen for them anyway and only have the capacity to withhold consent as long as they do not actually do so.

Beauchamp and Childress (2001) argue that popular and professional assumptions that high-risk decisions somehow require greater decision-making ability than those of less risk, have no foundation. Conversely, Buchanan and Brock (1989) are among those who suggest that the greater the risks or consequences of an action, the greater the level of competence required to make a decision. But it is not clear why it should necessarily follow that increased risk per se demands greater decision-making ability; Beauchamp and Childress argue that, on the contrary, low-risk decisions may demand more ability. They further suggest that it is the nature of the evidence determining competence that should vary in accordance with risk. So, perhaps it is the complexity of the decision and the individuals' capacity for understanding that is more important than the risks attached to it, but this distinction is not always made in practice. Fulbrook (1994) rightly acknowledges that an individual's competence is, in general, only called into question when the possible consequences of his/her decisions fail to conform to society's expectations.

Concerning authorisation of the practitioner by the patient client to carry out the recommended plan, it is important to note that there is no law of proxy or substituted judgement in the UK; in other words no adult may authorise treatment on behalf of another.

Adequacy of information

Once a more comprehensive conception of consent is accepted, so too are a number of specific responsibilities on the part of health care professionals. The process of obtaining consent must not only avoid untruths, respect individual autonomy, and promote informed decision-making, but also protect patients from harm, duress and anxiety (Cahill, 1998). Clearly, the information provided must be sufficient to allow an informed decision to be made, although some clinicians may think that they know what is best for their patients and may believe that giving too much information may not be in their best interests. However, this is an essentially erroneous assumption; as Kirby (1994, 446) rightly reiterates, patients are 'infinite in their variety and in their inclination to know medical detail and in their capacity to understand it, if explained'. Doctors and nurses are clearly accountable for their own competence and the quality of the information provided to a patient/client, but not for that patient/client's reaction to that information or any subsequent decision he or she makes. Doctors are, or should be, well informed about diagnostic techniques, the causes of disease, prognosis, treatment options, and preventive strategies, but only the patient/client knows about his or her experience of illness, their social circumstances, habits and behaviour, attitudes to risk, values, and preferences. Both types of knowledge are needed to manage illness successfully.

Although there is no requirement in English law that all possible side-effects of a treatment option must be outlined, the law in itself does not provide moral justification for omissions (Henry and Pashley, 1990). There are three competing standards against which the notion of adequate information can be assessed:

- The ***professional practice*** standard, established in Bolam in 1957 and upheld by Sidaway in 1985. Here adequate disclosure is determined by the customary practices of a professional community and it remains the dominant international standard

- The ***reasonable person*** standard holds that disclosure is adequate, if it is sufficient to permit a hypothetical 'reasonable' person to make an informed decision; this is the doctrine of informed consent that places the responsibility for adequate disclosure firmly with the clinician and, therefore, provides greater protection for patients' rights to self-determination than that defined in Bolam (Lindley, 1991). This is the alternative to the professional practice standard and is applied in around half of the states in the USA

- The ***subjective standard*** according to which the level of disclosure is considered adequate, if it is sufficient to enable the particular patient in question to make an informed decision. As both Black (1988) and Beauchamp and Childress (2001) acknowledge, perhaps this is the morally preferable standard of disclosure because of its greater recognition of individual patient needs.

The shift away from a paternalistic model in medical practice may have substantial effects on the law because, if all doctors are providing certain information, then a doctor who fails to do so may be deemed to be negligent. The law here is very closely tied to prevailing standards developed at the level of medical practice. Whatever standard of disclosure is adopted, health care professionals must assess patients' understanding of that information, and that brings home the importance of clarity of language. The requirements for informed consent require some level of patient engagement with decision-making, and the General Medical Council (1999) laid down stringent information requirements. The Department of Health are also now very clear about the extent of information provided to patients/clients. The Department of Health (Department of Health, 2001b) states that:

'Information about what the treatment will involve, its benefits and risks (including side-effects and complications) and the alternatives to the particular procedure

proposed, is crucial for patients when making up their
minds. The courts have stated that patients should be
told about 'significant risks which would affect the judge-
ment of a reasonable patient'... In addition, if patients
make clear they have particular concerns about certain
kinds of risk, you should make sure they are informed
about these risks, even if they are very small or rare.

It is important to emphasise that patients are not expected
to assume the level of knowledge and experience of health
professionals involved in their care in order to make a decision. But information given should include the purpose and
benefits of performing the intervention, the possible
options available, the discomfort and risks associated with
each option and the likely prognosis if nothing is done.
Giving patients such information may increase anxiety but,
equally, it may not. The principal weakness of the continued application of the professional practice standard is that
it assumes that doctors will always be able to accurately
predict that reaction when, clearly, that is not the case. The
important point is evidence of understanding.

Patients must have access to evidence-based information about proposed interventions, and accept responsibility for their decisions. Both Draper (1996a) and Madder
(1997) contend that assuming responsibility for oneself is
central to the exercise of autonomy; as Draper (1996a: 17)
puts it, 'where autonomous choice is exercised, responsibility follows'. In other words, exercising one's autonomy has a
price. Patients who autonomously refuse recommended
interventions must accept some measure of responsibility
for the outcome, which may be a deterioration in their
health or disability; i.e. they cannot refuse and then blame
others when things go wrong.

Who should obtain consent?

The Code of Conduct (NMC, 2002) places the responsibility for standards of care firmly in the hands of the individual practitioner. Particular reference should be paid to
clauses 2 and 3, i.e. those concerned with protecting

patients' interests and obtaining consent. Clause 3.10 states:

> *'usually, the individual performing a procedure should be the person to obtain the patient's or client's consent. In certain circumstances, you may seek consent on behalf of colleagues if you have been specially trained for that specific area of practice.'*

In law, the person performing the surgery or other procedure must be satisfied that the individual patient has the capacity to give that consent. Inappropriate delegation of consent processes may therefore invalidate consent.

In October 2002, the Department of Health's Consent Policy came into effect. This policy is slowly changing the custom and practice of obtaining patient consent for a range of interventions. The policy itself and the different forms required are all available on the Department of Health's website and the web addresses are to be found at the end of this chapter. In brief, for elective treatment requiring written authorisation, the consent process should have at least two stages: the provision of information, discussion of options, and initial decision (verbal); followed by confirmation that the patient/client still wants to go ahead. The Department of Health (2001b) states that the consent form should be used as a means of documenting both of the above stages and that the patient/client should have a copy of the page documenting the decision-making process. Patients/clients can sign the form at any appropriate point before the procedure to confirm that they wish to go ahead. This could be in the out-patients department, at a pre-admission clinic, or when they arrive for treatment. If a patient/client has signed the form in advance, a health professional involved in their care on the day (this can of course be a nurse) should ascertain whether or not they still wish to go ahead, and sign the form to confirm this. As the Department of Health makes clear, for consent to be valid, patients must be able to feel that refusal or a change of mind is possible. For that reason, the common practice of asking patients to sign a consent form after they have been prepared for treatment (in a gown, in bed) is no longer appropriate 'unless this is unavoidable because of the urgency of the patient's condition (Department of Health, 2001b).

Finally, how long does consent last? The answer is simple: for as long as the patient does not withdraw it. 'Patients may, if they wish, withdraw consent after they have signed a form: the signature is evidence of the process of consent-giving, not a binding contract' (Department of Health, 2001b).

In summary, consent processes must:

- be undertaken by appropriately trained practitioners
- assume patients are competent
- seek and respect patients' wishes
- ensure patients are adequately informed
- assess patients' understanding
- ensure patients' decisions are clearly articulated and free from coercion
- ensure that authorisation for treatment is documented appropriately, in line with local and national policy.

Consent, moral theory and the law

The principle of respect for autonomy

'Respect for autonomy is not a mere ideal in health care, it is a professional obligation. Autonomous choice is a right, not a duty of patients.'

(Beauchamp and Childress, 2001: 63)

Four intermediate moral principles are considered neutral in terms of underpinning medical ethics. One of these, respect for autonomy, defines the obligation to respect the autonomy of others (the other three principles being beneficence, non-maleficence and justice; see *Chapter One*). Beauchamp and Childress (2001) contend that these four principles have no rank order, only prima facie standing. In other words, we are obliged to abide by them all until the specific defining characteristics of a particular situation demand that one moral principle assumes precedence. However, it is unlikely that many doctors would put their skills in moral reasoning before those of clinical diagnosis and effective patient management. It is more likely that many would look to an 'all things considered, best interests' solution when faced with such a conflict. Seedhouse and Lovett (1992) suggest that most clinicians perceive medicine and ethics as being independent of each other, in that high quality clinical practice is their prime concern and attempts to act ethically are seen as a desirable yet essentially separate goal. But high quality clinical practice must, by definition, be ethically sound and the same is clearly so with nursing practice. So, to respect the autonomy of individual patients demands not only a positive attitude from doctors and nurses, but also respectful action. In other words, respecting an autonomous individual is to acknowledge that person's fundamental right to hold his/her own views, to make his/her own choices and to act in accord with his/her own personal values and beliefs.

The law and consent to treatment

Lord Donaldson makes it clear that the right to self-determination includes the right to refuse treatment:

> '*An adult patient who ... suffers from no mental incapacity has an absolute right to choose whether to consent to medical treatment, to refuse it or to choose one rather than another of the treatments being offered ... This right of choice is not limited to decisions which others might regard as sensible.*'

> (Re T [1992] 4 All ER 649, at 652–53)

Transgression of this general principle will give rise to two possible civil law actions, namely, battery or negligence. Even if a surgeon, for example, believes he or she has 'sufficient medical grounds' to proceed without consent, the law clearly states that treatment can be given without consent in the patient's best interests only in the case of necessity, emergency, or (if the patient is an adult) where the patient lacks capacity to consent (see section on competence). Without consent, any 'care', despite its best intentions and potentially beneficial outcomes, becomes 'unlawful touching' or trespass, which is in itself a civil wrong: 'the law requires that an adult patient who is mentally and physically capable of exercising a choice must consent if medical treatment of him is to be lawful' (Lord Donaldson [1992]: at 653). Any non-consensual contact (be it an injection, operation, insertion of a suppository, or whatever) constitutes the tort (i.e. civil wrong) of battery. The general principle of battery is as follows:

- The wrong lies in the undesired contact
- There must be physical contact
- The onus of proof is on the patient to establish that he/she did not consent.

So, an action in battery follows where there is no consent at all to the physical contact in question. In fact, relatively few cases have succeeded in English law. More recently there has been a shift away from battery to negligence. Here the question is less one of actual consent, but more one of the quality of the information that was given by doctors prior to gaining consent. It is also important to acknowledge that the same clearly applies to nurses obtaining consent for procedures they undertake. When a patient gives consent to the general nature of a procedure, but argues that the consent was flawed, an action may be brought in negligence. The general principle of negligence is that:

- A person has negligently breached a legal duty of care.
- He/she has by this breach caused a harm to others
- Therefore, he/she may be held liable.

All health care professionals owe a duty of care towards their patients, and a doctor's duty of care includes the duty to give careful advice and information upon which patients may reach an informed decision as to whether to accept or refuse surgery and other interventions. In the negligence action, the patient's claim is that the doctor failed to inform him/her of the risk that has in fact occurred, and had the doctor done so, he/she would not have consented to the procedure. Once more, the onus is on the patient to establish negligence.

The classic case is Bolam v Friern Hospital in 1957. Mr Bolam agreed to electro-convulsive therapy ECT to treat his depression and suffered fractures in the course of his treatment. At the time, muscle relaxants were not used as part of the sedation technique. Mr Bolam's doctor was aware of this risk, but did not tell him about it; Mr Bolam alleged that the doctor's failure to tell him of this risk was negligent. The judge found that the amount of information that was given to Mr Bolam was in accord with accepted medical practice in such cases (generally referred to as a 'responsible body of opinion'). In order to demonstrate negligence, Mr Bolam would have had to prove that, given better information, he would have refused consent. Not surprisingly, this is extremely difficult for a patient to prove. Even after 45 years, the 'Bolam test' is still utilised by the courts in judging whether or not a health professional has been negligent. Note that there may be a number of accepted ways to deal with a problem; just because you might not agree with the way a matter was handled does not automatically mean that there a was breach of duty of care.

Trust, best interests, and consent: An exercise

A 35-year-old woman is in hospital for a hysterectomy. On beginning the operation, the surgeon discovers that her uterus is enlarged and the most probable cause is pregnancy. He sends someone to look for the woman's husband in order to ask him whether the operation should go ahead. When he cannot be found, the surgeon goes ahead and performs the hysterectomy. The next day the woman is informed that an eleven-week foetus was removed along with her uterus; she is devastated. The couple have desperately wanted a child for some years and the woman only agreed to have a hysterectomy as she had been advised that the endometriosis from which she suffered had left her unable to conceive. This failure to conceive (along with other factors) had contributed to severe depression and had resulted in a failed suicide attempt. The surgeon is upset by the uproar. He agrees that, with the benefit of hindsight, maybe he took what has turned out to be the wrong decision. However, he is categorical that he acted in what he believed to be the woman's best interests. In particular, he states that given the woman's history of mental instability and her attempted suicide, he honestly believed that the shock of coming round from the anaesthetic to discover that (a) she had not had the operation, and (b) that she was pregnant, would have put her mental health at risk. He further argued that it was natural to assume that a woman who wanted children would not have consented to a hysterectomy.

Questions

1. On the basis of the facts before him in the operating theatre, do you think the surgeon was morally justified in going ahead with the operation?

2. What is the surgeon's position with regard to the termination of pregnancy?

3. Would it have made any difference if the woman's husband had been available to give the surgeon the go-ahead?

4. What might be said of the process of consent in this case?

5. Was this negligent action?
    (See end of chapter for answers)

Summary

Despite the law's continued support of the professional practice standard, the number of publications surrounding consent that have been published in the last few years are perhaps testament to increasing discomfort with this position (see, for example: Department of Health, 1997; GMC, 1999; MDU, 1996; NHSE, 1997). Doctors, on the one hand, appear to resent interference by the law into clinical practice, yet on the other resort to the law to force patient consent; this ambivalence both results in, and is perpetuated by, defensive practice and inadequate disclosure of information. And patients, who have had the temerity to disagree with expert medical opinion, have paid the price (Cahill, 1999).

This chapter has explored some of the key ethical and legal issues underpinning the concept of valid consent. An important element of more recent health service reform has been the increased emphasis on patients' rights, choices and involvement in decision-making regarding their care (Cahill and Jackson, 1997); a development that is both legitimate and well overdue. Protocols for consent must take this significant shift in authority into account. Valid consent to surgery is both an expression of respect for autonomy and a legal safeguard for patients best interests; it is far from being just a signature on a form.

References

Beauchamp TL, Childress JF (2001) *Principles of Biomedical Ethics*, 5th edn. Oxford University Press, New York

Black, D (1988) Guidelines or gumption? The role of medical responsibility: a view from the profession. In: Hirsch SR, Harris J, eds. *Consent and the Incompetent Patient: Ethics, Law and Medicine*. Gaskell, London

Buchanan AE, Brock DW (1989) *Deciding for Others: The Ethics of Surrogate Decision-Making*. Cambridge University Press, Cambridge

Cahill H (1999) An Orwellian scenario: court ordered caesarean section and women's autonomy. *Nurs Ethics* **6**(6): 492–503

Cahill H (1998) Moral and legal aspects of consent in day surgery. *J One-Day Surg* **8**(2): 3–5

Cahill H, Jackson I (1997) *Day Surgery: Principles and Nursing Practice*. Bailliere Tindall, London

Department of Health (2001a) Reference guide to consent for examination or treatment: http://www.doh.gov.uk/consent/refguide.pdf

Department of Health (2001b) Good practice in consent implementation guide: consent to examination or treatment: www.doh.gov.uk/consent/implementationguide.pdf

Department of Health (1997) *A Guide to Consent for Examination or Treatment*. The Stationery Office, London

Dimond B (1995) *Legal Aspects of Nursing,* 2nd edn. Prentice-Hall, London

Downie RS, Calman KC (1994) *Healthy Respect: Ethics in Healthcare,* 2nd edn. Oxford University Press, Oxford

Draper H (1996a) Women, forced caesareans and antenatal responsibilities. J Med Ethics **22**: 327–33

Draper H (1996b) Consent in childbirth. In: Frith L, ed. *Ethics and Midwifery: Issues in Contemporary Practice.* Butterworth Heinemann, Oxford

Dworkin G (1988) *The Theory and Practice of Autonomy*. Cambridge University Press, Cambridge

Dyer O (2002) GMC reprimands consultant for terminating pregnancy without consent. *Br Med J* **324**: 1354

Faulder C (1985) *Whose body is it? The Troubling Issue of Informed Consent*. Virago Press, London

Fulbrook P (1994) Assessing mental competence of patients and relatives. *J Adv Nurs* **20**: 457–61

General Medical Council (1999) *Seeking Patients' Consent: The Ethical Considerations.* GMC, London:

Gillon R (1986) *Philosophical Medical Ethics*. John Wiley, Chichester

Henry IC, Pashley G (1990) *Health Ethics*. Quay, Lancaster

Kennedy I (1992) Consent to treatment: The capable person. In: Dyer C, ed. *Doctors, Patients and the Law*. Blackwell Scientific, Oxford

Kessel AS (1994) On failing to understand informed consent. *Br J Hosp Med* **52**(5): 235–38

Kirby M (1994) Consent and the doctor-patient relationship. In: Gillon R, ed. *Principles of Health Care Ethics*. John Wiley & Sons, Chichester

Lindley R (1991) Informed consent and the ghost of Bolam. In: Brazier M, Lobjoit M, eds. *Protecting the Vulnerable. Autonomy and Consent in Health Care*. Routledge, London

Madder H (1997) Existential autonomy: why patients should make their own choices. *J Med Ethics* **23**: 221–25

Mason JK, McCall-Smith RA (1994) *Law and Medical Ethics*, 4th edn. Butterworth, London

McLean S, Maher G (1993) *Medicine, Morals and the Law*. Oxford University Press, Oxford

McMillan RC (1995) Responsibility to or for in the physician-patient relationship? *J Med Ethics* **21**(2): 112–15

Medical Defence Union (1996) *Consent to Treatment*. MDU, London

Montgomery J (2002) *Health Care Law*, 2nd edn. Oxford University Press, Oxford

NHS E (1997) *Consent to Treatment—Summary of Legal Rulings*; Executive Letter EL (97) 32. NHSE, Leeds

Nursing and Midwifery Council (2002) *Code of Conduct*. NMC, London

Robinson J (1995) Informed refusal. *Br J Midwifery* **3**(11): 616–17

Seedhouse D, Lovett L (1992) *Practical Medical Ethics*. John Wiley and Son, Chichester

Worthington R (2002) Clinical issues on consent: some philosophical concerns. *J Med Ethics* **28**: 377–80

Further reading

British Medical Association (2001) *Consent Toolkit*. Available at: http://web.bma.org.uk/public/pubother

Department of Health (2001c) Model policy for consent to examination or treatment: www.doh.gov.uk/consent/modelconsentpolicy.doc

Department of Health (2001) HSC 2001/023 *Good Practice in Consent: Achieving the NHS Plan Commitment to Patient-Centred Consent Practice.* Department of Health, London

Department of Health (2001) Seeking Consent—Working with Children: www.doh.gov.uk/consent/childrensguidance.pdf

Department of Health (2001) Seeking Consent—Working with Older people: www.doh.gov.uk/consent/olderpeople.pdf

Legal cases

Bolam v Friern Hospital [1957] 2 All ER 118

Re C (Adult: Refusal of Treatment) [1994] 1 All ER 819

Re T (Adult: Refusal of Treatment) [1992] 4 All ER 649

Sidaway v Board of Governors of the Bethlem Royal Hospital and Maudsley Hospital [1985] 1 All ER 643

Web sites

British Medical Association Ethics pages: web.bma.org.uk/public/ethics.nsf/webguidlinesvw? open view

Human Rights Act www.hmso.gov.uk/acts/acts1998/19980042.htm

BMJ Collection—Consent www.bmj.com/cgi/collec-tion/informed_consent

The consent forms

Patient agreement to investigation or treatment: www.doh.gov.uk/consent/consentform1.doc

Parental agreement to investigation or treatment for a child or young person: www.doh.gov.uk/consent/consentform2.doc

Patient/parental agreement to investigation or treatment (procedures where consciousness not impaired): www.doh.gov.uk/consent/consentform3.doc

Form for adults who are unable to consent to investigation or treatment: www.doh.gov.uk/consent/consentform4.doc

Answers to exercise

a)   no—the woman was not bleeding, it was not an emergency, so he couldn't claim necessity as defence. He knew how much she wanted a baby. He should have stopped, returned her to the ward and discussed his findings with her and let the woman herself make the decision; she was autonomous and competent;

b)   strictly unlawful—done without consent—though he was acquitted of illegally procuring an abortion in 1995;

c)   no—remember the position regarding proxy consent;

d)   Poor—the possibility of pregnancy was obviously never discussed or documented;

e)   it sound like it was but.... Remember the courts acceptance of the professional practice standard—there may be a number of accepted ways to deal with a case such as this; just because you might not agree with the way the surgeon acted does not automatically mean that there a was breach of duty of care. He was able to bring expert witness to testify that a significant body of medical opinion would have acted in the same way.

Before you lay all the blame at the feet of the surgeon, remember that there were probably four or five other people in the theatre including nurses, who did nothing to stop the surgery going ahead. Remember this when someone tells you about the role of the nurse as patient/client advocate. Incidentally, the surgeon (a consultant obstetrician and gynaecologist) was severely reprimanded by the General Medical Council in 2002 (the year after he retired) for terminating the pregnancy without consent (see Dyer, 2002).

6

RESTRICTIVE PHYSICAL INTERVENTIONS

M Wolverson

Introduction

This chapter will offer an exploration of the ethical issues associated with the use of restrictive physical interventions in health and social care settings. The decision to use a restrictive physical intervention is taken by a person or persons other than the recipient of the intervention and, in most instances, without their consent. So restrictive physical intervention is apparently at odds with the autonomy of the person who is subject to such interventions. The ethical dilemmas that arise as a result are, in the main, a result of the conflicting ethical theories of autonomy and paternalism. The dilemmas resulting from the use of restrictive physical interventions are further complicated by a significant amount of evidence suggesting such restrictive physical interventions can have deleterious outcomes, are of doubtful benefit, and can increase the risk of death (Evans *et al*, 2003). The complex ethical underpinning of the use of restrictive physical interventions is also influenced by the notion of 'best interest', and the desire to protect the individual from harm and to prevent him/her from harming others. Thus the main aims of this chapter are:

- to explore (partly by the use of four case studies) the ethical dilemmas that commonly emanate from the use of restrictive physical interventions
- to explain how an understanding of ethics can inform the decision-making process(es) that impact on restrictive physical interventions

- to demonstrate how and when the use of restrictive physical interventions may be ethically justified.

In pursuit of these aims, the chapter will define what is meant by restrictive physical interventions. This requires discussion of the concept of personhood and the 'setting' conditions which increase the likelihood of restrictive physical interventions being used.

Definitions

It is helpful for care staff to have an understanding of what may constitute a restrictive physical intervention. Some interventions may not be perceived to be restrictive, as a result of which, care staff may sometimes engage in physical interventions without realising that they are doing so. This can have legal as well as ethical implications. It should be noted that services may employ other words and/or terminology to indicate what may be included within the broad heading of 'restrictive physical interventions'. In some care settings, particularly those designed to care for people with behavioural problems, the approach termed 'Control and Restraint' or 'C and R' is often used synonymously with 'restrictive physical interventions'. This can be confusing as the term is used to denote many other forms of restrictive intervention. Attempts have been made to offer comprehensive definitions, for example, Retsas (1998: 186) states that physical and/or mechanical restraints are, 'any device material or equipment attached to or near a person's body and which cannot be controlled or easily removed by the person and which deliberately prevents or is deliberately intended to prevent a person's free body movement to a position of choice and/or a person's normal access to their body'.

This definition is useful, however the term 'restrictive physical interventions' includes other practices. The Department of Health (2002)—with reference to people with learning disabilities, although the examples are generalisable—expand on the above definition by also indicating that bodily contact (examples range from holding a person's hand to prevent them from hitting out, to control and restraint) and the manipulation of the environment (examples range from the use of baffle locks, to seclusion) can be interpreted as restrictive physical interventions. It is important that care staff are aware that the use of medication which compromises the individual's ability to exercise freewill should be viewed as a restrictive physical intervention (Brennan, 1999). It is apparent that some interventions, such as control and restraint, are quite clearly extremely restrictive, whereas others, such as baffle locks, may not immediately appear to be so. This is important as there is widespread evidence suggesting that some mechanisms—for example, wheelchairs—which are usually not perceived to be restrictive devices, can be effectively used as such (Simmons *et al*, 1995). Clarke and Bright (2002) comment that there are insidious and subtle ways in which a person's liberty and autonomy can be interfered with in care settings, for example, reducing the heating in particular rooms to discourage their use. Horsburgh (2003) comments that, if items of apparatus necessary for an autonomous lifestyle, such as walking aids, are made unavailable to an individual, the outcome is de facto restraint.

This discussion of what can constitute restrictive physical interventions has demonstrated that it is a generic term used to cover a spectrum of interventions and practices. Although the term covers a range of interventions, they share a commonality in that they all in some way interfere to some degree with a person's autonomy and in so doing create ethical dilemmas.

The concept of personhood and 'setting' conditions

There is much evidence to suggest that some groups of people, either throughout the whole of their life or temporarily, are more likely to be subject to restrictive physical interventions than others, due to their perceived health status (Craig, 1999; Irving, 2002; Mion *et al*, 1989). Restrictive physical interventions have been associated with the following groups of people and setting conditions:

- Older people
- Having difficulty in giving or being unable to give consent
- Morbidity
- Lengthy periods in care settings
- Presence of mental ill health or perceived 'abnormality'
- Presence of organic brain syndrome
- Surgery
- Physical dependency
- Decreased cognitive status
- Increased severity of illness
- Being male within the context of other setting conditions
- Disorientation
- People with learning disabilities
- Those perceived to be a risk to self or others
- Presence of medical devices (e.g. catheters, IV tubing, nasogastric tubes)
- Behavioural problems.

These 'setting' conditions can be seen to alter the perception of the 'personhood' of the individuals to whom they apply. The concept of personhood is extremely important in that it is a highly significant factor in the ethical conflict between autonomy and paternalism underlying the use of restrictive physical interventions. The definition and understanding of what constitutes a 'person' is also extremely important because it can influence the way that individual care workers, staff teams, communities and society in general treat those whose personhood is compromised. Ethicists and philosophers have contemplated the qualities that define a 'person' throughout history and a consensus opinion is that the key element of being a person is rationality. Johnstone (1989) has expanded on this and states that personhood is defined by the following criteria:

- Being conscious of objects and events that are external and/or internal to the being and particularly the ability to feel pain
- The ability to reason and have the capacity to solve problems
- The capacity for self–motivated activity that is relatively independent of genetic or direct external control
- The ability to communicate, by whatever means, a variety of messages that could cover an indefinite range of topics
- Having a concept of one's self, and a sense of self-awareness.

It is a plausible assumption that a combination of the setting factors outlined above and an absence of some of the criteria of personhood can lead to care staff perceiving those affected as having difficulty in exercising freewill or being incapable of doing so at all. Irving (2002) has explained that such a view can lead to the stigmatisation of those so perceived and lead to their infantalisation and objectification. This process can lead to care staff deciding to act in paternalistic ways at the expense of the person's autonomy. It is a commonly held view that autonomy and self-determination are principles that should be respected by others. However, the right to self-govern is often denied to those subject to restrictive physical interventions due to the setting conditions outlined above.

A further area for consideration is the potential antagonism between rights and responsibilities. Curtin and Flaherty (1982) maintain that duties, obligations to others and responsibility are the 'mirror images' of individual rights. Curtin and Flaherty go on to say that each fundamental right, such as the right to self-govern, carries with it 'corollary' duties that affect both the individual and others.

In ethical terms, this is referred to as 'logical and moral correlativity'. In relation to the justification of restrictive physical interventions, logical and moral correlativity could apply in situations where a person forfeits his/her right to autonomous action if it would result in harm to others and the only way to prevent this is the use of restraint. The right to self-govern is also potentially compromised by the notions of 'duty of care' and 'best interests', both of which can lead to care workers acting in a paternalistic manner at the expense of autonomy. The Nursing and Midwifery Council Code of Professional Conduct states: 'You have a duty of care to your patients and clients, who are entitled to receive safe and competent care' (NMC, 2002: 3).

Although the code of conduct applies specifically to nurses, the principles that underpin it and the potential outcomes are generalisable to other groups of care workers. It may well be that nurses struggle to balance the autonomous wishes of patients (which are also covered by the NMC Code of Conduct in point 3.2) that may seem irrational against their interpretation of 'the duty of care'. This may compel the nurse to act in paternalistic ways that she construes to be in the patient's best interests even if it is against his/her expressed will. Care staff often explain the use of restrictive physical interventions by maintaining that they are acting in a person's best interests. This assertion may justify their decisions, but it is sometimes the case that restrictive physical interventions are used without ascertaining what the person's best interests actually are. Within the care setting, the concept of 'best interests' can sometimes be used in a casual, facile and disingenuous way. It is also the case that restrictive physical interventions can be used in the best interest of the service provider and care staff, as opposed to patient. Artnak (1997) has commented that the notion of what constitutes best interest in a nursing environment can be based on the medical model of care with the intention being the preservation of life and the relief of suffering. This may be a laudable goal, but it could interfere with the autonomous decision-making of the individual and as such can be seen to be ethically questionable. There can be a presumption that care staff understand the meaning of 'best interest' when in fact no clear consensus exists in practice. Some clarity with regard to the considerations that should be taken into account when attempting to decide what may be in the best interests of an individual has been provided by The Law Commission (1995):

- the ascertainable past and present wishes and feelings of the person concerned and the factors the person would consider if he/she were able to do so
- the need to permit and encourage the person to participate as fully as possible in anything done for, and any decision affecting, him or her
- the views of other people whom it is appropriate and practical to consult about the person's wishes and feelings and what would be in his or her best interests
- whether the purpose for which any action or decision is required can be as effectively achieved in a manner less restrictive of the person's freedom of action.

The final point is interesting in that it suggests that the use of restrictive physical interventions should be a last resort after alternatives have been considered. There is a consensual view that this should be the case and guidance for the use of them (see, for example, Department of Health, 2002) recommends that alternatives are sought and yet the prevalence of their use remains high (Craig, 1997). This raises the suspicion that, in some instances, alternatives to restrictive physical interventions have not been fully explored and that this, in itself, is ethically unjustifiable and increases the number and complexity of dilemmas encountered by care staff. It is evident that care-givers can experience confusion engendered by the conflict between the obligation to fulfil their 'duty of care' while acting in the 'best interests' of those they care for in relation to the use of restrictive physical interventions. The case studies included in this chapter will explore this ambivalence further. Although the central ethical conflict in health care is almost always that of paternalism versus autonomy, all other ethical theories underpin this antagonism. There are sub-relationships between them and each will now be discussed in turn, with an outline of how they either justify or mitigate against both paternalism or autonomy.

Ethical theories and restrictive physical interventions

All the chapters in this book can give further depth to the issues covered in this chapter; however, *Chapter One* should be read in conjunction with this chapter as it explains in more detail the main ethical theories outlined below. The following information is intended to clarify how key ethical theories might be used to justify the use of restrictive physical interventions. It is possible that some ethical theories can both support and argue against the use of restrictive physical interventions.

Autonomy

An understanding of the importance of the rights of autonomy, freewill and self-determination is a prerequisite of exploring the ethical dilemmas associated with restrictive physical interventions. This is largely because there is a consensual agreement that self-government is self-evidently a fundamental human right. Any interference with a person's autonomy can be seen to be unethical. It is inevitable that restrictive physical interventions will, to some extent, compromise an individual's autonomy. The understanding that the use of restrictive physical interventions interferes with this basic human right and that this is ethically questionable has led to the development of a plethora of laws, policies, guidelines and procedures that attempt to balance the right of the individual to self-determination against the potential necessity of restrictive physical intervention.

Paternalism

The ethical counterpoint of autonomy is paternalism. The use of restrictive physical interventions is intrinsically paternalistic. Kay (1994) argues that, in purely ethical terms, paternalism is unethical as it negates freewill. This is the central ethical conflict in the provision of care services as there are situations in which a paternalistic intervention is a 'lesser of two evils', i.e. the least worse option. Care staff need to conduct a mental balancing act that weighs the freewill of the individual against the potential outcomes of intervention, which can be either negative, positive or a mixture of the two. Care staff should be aware that non-intervention is in itself a kind of intervention and that, in some instances, some form of restrictive measures will be the only valid option available to them and that this can be ethically justified. The notion of 'moral correlativity' (as outlined earlier) can contribute to a justification of a paternalistic use of restrictive physical interventions in that the right to autonomy can be seen to be dependant on the responsibility not to jeopardise the rights and well-being of others. An example of this is provided by the rare, but sometimes necessary accommodation of people, who present a persistent threat of aggression, away from those to whom they present the danger.

Beneficence/non-maleficence

The concepts of beneficence and non-maleficence contribute to the dilemmas emanating from the use of restrictive physical interventions in that any intervention should result in more good and less harm than non-intervention. There is an assumption that care-givers have a wish to operate from this ethical underpinning and it is strongly associated with the notion of 'best interest' outlined earlier in the chapter. An example of this is provided by minimum restraint being used (holding the arms of the person) to obtain a blood sample to test for anti-convulsant levels from a person with learning disability and who cannot give consent (see *Case Study 2*).

Consequentialism/utilitarianism

Any debate regarding the use of restrictive physical interventions must be informed by a consideration of the consequences of both implementing and not implementing the intervention. Consideration should be given to the potential short- and long-term outcomes of any restrictive intervention on the individual concerned, significant others and those using the restrictive intervention. A restrictive physical intervention is more likely to be ethically justified if the consequences of doing so result in more positive than negative outcomes. An example of this is provided by the use of baffle locks in a care home for people with dementia. The use of baffle locks can obviously be perceived to be a restrictive measure that compromises an individual's autonomy; however, the 'wandering' behaviour sometimes associated with dementia could result in negative conse-quences if a person is not prevented by the baffle locks from leaving the home and encountering potentially dangerous situations (see *Case Study 3*).

Deontology

Deontological ethical theory is concerned with obliga-tions and duties. In most care settings, care staff would con-sider that their duty of care is related to the individuals for whom they care and that they have an obligation to main-tain their autonomy. In relation to restrictive physical interventions, this can be interpreted in two ways. Firstly, a care giver may consider that his/her duty of care over-rides, in some instances, the freewill of the person subject to an intervention. An example of this would be a decision to give potentially life-saving treatment to a person who is incapacitated that interfered with the recipients freewill by involving some form of restrictive intervention. Secondly, care staff may consider they have more of an obligation and duty of care to those who may be harmed, if a restrictive intervention were not implemented. An example of this would be the forced removal of flammable materials from a person with a personality disorder and a history of arson in a psychiatric treatment and assessment unit. This restrictive action obviously compromises the freewill of the individual, but it demonstrates that the duty and obligation to protect the well-being of others has been achieved.

Case studies

An understanding of ethical theory provides a framework for decision-making in practice. This framework can be used by care staff to justify and account for the decisions they take in practice relating to the dilemmas associated with restrictive physical interventions. A dilemma is different from a problem in that problems are solvable. Ethical dilemmas require the application of a framework of ethical theories, so that the most beneficial and least harmful outcome(s) can be achieved. The following case studies will give examples of some of the ethical dilemmas encountered as a result of restrictive physical interventions, and how an ethical framework can support judicious and pragmatic decision-making.

Case Study 1: control and restraint

As mentioned earlier in the chapter, an approach to managing aggression in some care environments is the sanctioned use of control and restraint. This approach should only be used by care staff who have been trained in the procedure. Its use is contentious and some commentators have opposed it. Hopton (1995) maintains that it is an inherently dangerous practice that risks injury and death. Malasiotis (1995) and McDougall (1996) both stress that huge psychological harm can be caused by control and restraint and McDougall goes on to say that restraint can be used as a punishment and not as a last resort. It is evident that the use of control and restraint is a practice that temporarily prevents a person from exercising freewill; however, there is an understanding that this is necessary in some circumstances (Department of Health, 2002):

John has been diagnosed as having a personality disorder. He has had periods of disturbed and aggressive behaviour resulting in him being detained under a section of the Mental Health Act (1983). He lives in a specialist unit with eight people with similar histories. On occasions, there have been antagonisms between John and the some of the other people in the unit. These antagonisms have resulted in John breaking furniture and attempting to use pieces of it as weapons with which to attack people. On these occasions John is restrained.

The ethical dilemmas arising from this situation are clearly that John's autonomy is negated in a paternalistic manner. Beauchamp and Childress (1989) question the extent to which a person (such as John) who is detained can exercise freewill, autonomy and self-determinism. The act of physically restraining John further denies him his autonomy. Clearly, there are ethical conflicts in this situation. From the ethical standpoint of beneficence, it could be argued that restraint is not of benefit to John as it could result in physical harm and psychological damage and this could be perceived to be a malevolent act. A consequentialist ethical stance would, to some degree, demonstrate that some potential outcomes of the restraint could be negative for John. A deontological perspective could bring into question whether care staff had abrogated their duty of care to John by intervening in a way that is potentially harmful to him.

The ethical counterpoint to these concerns is one of 'benevolent paternalism' supported by other ethical theories. The concept of beneficence and non-maleficence can be used to support the restraint as it prevents those around John from being harmed. Consequentialism and utilitarianism can also support this intervention as the consequences of not intervening could result in significant harm to others, and most benefit accrues from the intervention. From a deontological perspective, care staff have an obligation and duty to care for, not only John, but the other people in their care. Thus an ethical framework can be applied to the dilemmas associated with control and restraint and aid decision-making.

Case Study 2: invasive procedures

David has a severe learning disability, cerebral palsy and epilepsy. His epilepsy is relatively well-controlled by the use of anti-convulsant medication; however, David does have seizures on occasions that can result in status epilepticus and this could ultimately result in his death. In order that David has a therapeutic dosage of anti-convulsants and so that they do not reach toxic levels, it is periodically necessary to check the levels in his blood. It is consensually agreed that David does not have the capacity to consent to a blood test; however, it does seem that David implies that he may not wish to allow his blood to be taken through his body language. David appears afraid of needles and he becomes tense when he is approached by the care team in a first attempt at taking blood. This issue was discussed by the care team and it was proposed by the responsible medical officer that David's arm might need to be held during the procedure, but he would be constantly reassured. It was also suggested that David could be given a small dose of diazepam four hours before having his blood taken. It should be noted that when an individual lacks the capacity to give consent, then the health professional responsible for that person's care is responsible for deciding if an intervention is in the person's best interests.

The care team responsible for David's care were concerned about this situation. Their concerns centred around the ethical conflict of paternalism and autonomy. The staff involved in caring for David were cognisant of their duty of care to him and their caring ethos is based on a respect for his autonomy. It was evident that if a decision was taken to hold David's arm while blood was taken, this would constitute a minimum level of restraint and it would compromise David's freewill. When applying the principles of benevolence and consequentialism to this situation, staff were concerned that the outcome may not be entirely beneficial for David as he may become stressed by the procedure and the trusting relationship that had developed with care staff could be damaged.

The staff team were also concerned about the potential outcomes that may occur if the test does not take place. The test could be seen to be justifiable as the potential outcomes of not taking the blood could be interpreted as being contrary to the duty of care. The care staff have an obligation to act in David's 'best interests' and they could plausibly claim to be doing so in taking the blood as not to do so could have significantly negative outcomes. This stance is supported by the Department of Health (2001), a reading of which would help to clarify and add depth to this case study. From a utilitarian perspective, the test could be seen to be justified as the negative consequences of taking the blood could be perceived to be superseded by those of not doing so; it is likely that a greater good will arise from taking the blood than from not doing so.

Case Study 3: controlling the environment

There is much evidence to suggest that that older people with dementia can have behavioural problems (Flick and Foreman, 2000; Ignatavicius, 1999; Rateau, 2000). Health and social care staff have attempted to control such behaviour by using restraints and Whitehead *et al* (1997) have demonstrated that 12.5% of older hospitalised people are subject to physical and chemical restraint. Ashcroft-Simpson (1999) lists the practices that have been used as restraint and these include positioning people on tip-back, or low bean bag style chairs and the use of apparatus with trays or tables that prevent people from getting up. Ashcroft- Simpson also report that people have been restrained by tying limbs to furniture. It has been indicated by various commentators that the prevalence of such overtly restraining methods has been greatly reduced due to human rights legislation and litigation (Godkin and Onyskiw, 1999) and a belief that they are both ineffective and dangerous (Evans *et al*, 2003). While the use of overt forms of restrictive physical interventions has decreased, the use of other restrictive practices, such as the locking of doors and the use of baffle locks to prevent people from wandering, continues (Strathen, 1992).

Holly House provides care for twenty people who have dementia. Most but not all of them display the wandering behaviour associated with dementia. Some of these people will wander from Holly House and encounter dangerous situations, such as busy roads. It has become common practice at Holly House to lock the main entry doors and to control movement within the building by the use of strategically placed baffle locks. This practice has been questioned by a visitor to Holly House who has complained to the local inspectorate about the infringement of her father's human rights.

This situation once again revolves around the central ethical conflict between autonomy and paternalism. As discussed earlier in the chapter, any situation that interferes with a person's autonomy is ethically questionable. Clearly, the autonomy of the people at Holly House is severely compromised by the locking of doors, which is a paternalistic act. This denial of freewill can have negative outcomes, such as psychological damage, frustration and a decrease in self-esteem (Sullivan-Marx, 1995). From the ethical perspective, beneficence is compromised as some harm can accrue as a result. A consequentialist view would suggest that the outcome(s) of this practice is negative. A deontological stance would question whether the care staff's duty of care is jeopardised by this infringement of freewill.

Those ethical theories that can be used to question the practice of locking doors can also be employed to justify it. From the deontological perspective, the duty of care held by the care staff dictates that they should keep the people in their care safe and the locking of doors is a way of doing this. A consequentialist view may indicate that this practice has potentially more positive than negative outcomes in that it can prevent harm. The notion of beneficence could also be used to justify this practice as it may result in more good than harm. The utilitarian stance could also support the decision to regulate free movement as it is likely to result in more benefit than harm. The ethical arguments that support this interference with self-government combine to possibly justify 'benevolent paternalism'. Horsborough (2003) has argued that it may be justifiable to override a person's (with dementia and wandering behaviour) autonomy as he/she may lack the insight to understand the potentially damaging outcomes of his/her actions. In such circumstances, it may be that, after careful consideration, a benevolently paternalistic action is ethically justified. It is worthy of note that the Department of Health's Social Services Inspectorate (1995) recognised that balances need to be applied between needs, wishes and the freedom of choice of individuals.

Case Study 4: insidious restraint

Bennett *et al* (1997) discuss the widespread use of insidious restraints that involve restriction and coercion relating to personal choice and lifestyle. An example of this is when the resources needed for a person to express choice are denied to him/her.

> Susan has a mild learning disability and cerebral palsy and this has resulted in her being dependent on care staff in relation to being able to access social activities. She lives in a care home with six other people who have similar needs. Susan has always enjoyed going to church on Sunday mornings, but she can only get there if taken by the staff responsible for her care using the home's mini-bus. The other people who live with Susan prefer to sleep late on Sundays rather than go to church. They also use the mini-bus on Sundays to go out to engage in social activities which are usually suggested by staff. Staff are aware that Susan is distressed because she cannot go to church, but feel that the use of the home's resources (the staff and the bus) are better employed by current arrangements.

This situation clearly prevents Susan from exercising her freewill and while it may not appear as overtly restrictive as some forms of restraint, the outcomes are the same. From the viewpoint of beneficence and non-maleficence, the care staff may believe that they are not doing anything that will significantly harm Susan while also being aware that their actions will not benefit her. Similarly, a consequentialist view could conclude that, seemingly little harm may result from this arrangement and that other people benefit from it. As regards the deontological perspective, the duty of care to Susan is being disregarded, although it could be argued that this is because of competing obligations to others.

It is apparent that the decision of the care staff is driven by utilitarian principles in that they believe maximum benefit will result from this arrangement. But their decision is obviously paternalistic in that it denies Susan the right to exercise freewill. Situations that arise from the apportioning of finite resources often result in ethical dilemmas that stem from the denial of freewill. Services will generally act in ways that can be interpreted as being beneficial to the majority at the possible expense of the autonomy of individuals or a minority. The ethical justification for this is highly questionable. Rather than focussing on individual dilemmas, it could be argued that it is the under-resourcing of care services that is the cause of such dilemmas and that it is this issue that is, in itself, unethical.

Summary

This chapter has offered an introductory exploration of the ethical dilemmas associated with the use of restrictive physical interventions in health and social care settings. Ashton (1997: 8) commented that there is 'inevitable conflict between empowerment and protection, because you cannot protect without taking away some of the rights you seek to preserve'. Ashton alludes to the central ethical conflict that has been discussed in this chapter—that of autonomy versus paternalism. It was demonstrated that other ethical theories can be used to examine ethical dilemmas. It was made evident that health and social care staff can use ethical theory to help them in their decision-making in practice. It was demonstrated that it is sometimes necessary for practitioners to conduct a mental balancing act, informed by ethical awareness and the notions of personhood and best interests. It is hoped that the processes outlined in this chapter will enable care staff to feel more confident with the decisions they may be involved in relating to the use of restrictive physical interventions.

References

Artnak KE (1997) Informed consent in the elderly: assessing decisional capacity. *Seminars Periop.Nursing* **6**(1): 59–64

Ashcroft-Simpson S (1999) Nurses and the use of restraint. *Educat Ageing* **14**(1)

Ashton G (1997) The legal dilemmas of risk and rights. *Eagle,* April/May 4–8

Beauchamp TL, Childress JF (1989) *Principles of Biomedical Ethics.* Oxford University Press, Oxford

Bennet G, Kingston P, Penhale B (1997) *Dimensions of Elder Abuse: Perspectives for the Practitioner.* Macmillan, Basingstoke

Brennan S (1999) Dangerous liaisons. *Nursing Times* **95**(44): 30–32

Clarke A, Bright L (2002) *Showing Restraint: Challenging the Use of Restraint in Care Homes.* Counsel and Care, London

Craig D (1999) Mechanically restraining the ill and elderly: Ethical problems and proposals. *Bioethics Update* **15**(4): (December 1999) Loma Linda University

Curtin L (1982) What are human rights. In:Curtin L, Flaherty JM, eds. *Nursing Ethics, Theories and Pragmatics.* Prentice Hall Publications, London

Department of Health (2002) Guidance for Restrictive Physical Interventions: How to Provide Safe Services for People with Learning Disabilities and Autistic Spectrum Disorder. Available at: *www.doh.gov.uk/learningdisabilities*

Department of Health (2001) Seeking Consent: Working with People with Learning Disabilities. Available at: *www.doh.gov.uk/consent*

Department of Health (Social Services Inspectorate (1995) *Messages for Staff from Inspections of Local Authority Care Homes.* HMSO, London

Evans D, Wood J, Lambert L (2003) Patient injury and physical restraint devices:a systematic review. *J Adv Nurs* **41**(3): 274–82

Flick D, Foreman M (2000) Consequences of not recognising delirium superimposed on dementia in hospitalised elderly individuals. *J Gerontol Nurs* **26**: 30–40

Godkin MD, Onyskiw JE (1999) A systematic overview of interventions to reduce physical restraint use in long-term care settings. *The Online Journal of Knowledge Synthesis for Nursing* 6(6)

Hopton J (1995) Control and restraint in contemporary psychiatric nursing: some ethical considerations. *J Adv Nurs* **22**: 110–15

Horsburgh D (2003) The ethical implications and legal aspects of patient restraint. *Nursing Times* **99**(6): 26–27

Ignatavicius D (1999) Resolving the delirium dilemma. *Nursing* **29**(10): 41–46

Irving K (2002) Governing the conduct of conduct: are restraints inevitable. *J Adv Nurs* **40**(4): 405–12

Johnstone MJ (1989) *Bioethics: A Nursing Perspective.* Saunders, Marrickville

Kay B (1994) People with learning disabilities. In: Tschudin V, ed. *Ethics:Nursing People with Special Needs,* Part 11. .Scutari Press, Harrow

Law Commission Report No. 231(summary) (1995) *Mental Incapacity.* London

Malasitotis A (1995) Use of Physical Restraints. *Br J Nurs* **4**(3): 31–39

McDougall T (1996) Physical restraint: a review of the literature. *Psychiatric Care* **3**(4): 132–38

Mental Health Act 1983. HMSO, London.

Mion LC, Frengley JD, Jakovic CA, Marino JA (1989) A further exploration of the use of physical restraints in hospitalised patients. *J Am Geriatric Soc* **37**: 949–56

Nursing and Midwifery Council (2002) Code of Professional Conduct. Available at: *www.nmc-uk.org*

Rateau MR (2000) Confusion and aggression in restrained elderly persons undergoing hip repair surgery. *Appl Nurs Res J* **13**: 50–54

Retsas AP (1998) Survey findings describing the use of physical restraints in nursing homes in Victoria, Autstralia. *Int J Nurs Stud* **35**: 184–91

Simmons SF *et al* (1995) Wheelchairs as mobility restraints: predictors of wheelchair activity in non-ambulatory nursing home residents. *J Am Geriatr Soc* **43**: 384–88

Strathen D (1992) *What If They Hurt Themselves?* Counsel and Care, London

Sullivan-Marx EM (1995) Psychological responses to physical restraint use in adults. *J Gerontol Nurs* **20**(12): 19–24

Whitehead C, Finucane P, Henschke P, Nicholson F (1997) Use of patient restraints in four Australian teaching hospitals. *J Qual Clin Pract* **17**: 131–36

7

RESEARCH ETHICS

A Richardson and L Sitton-Kent

Introduction

For many people, the view that research is an important component of nursing is one that may not always be obvious. However, in the twenty-first century it is clearly no longer acceptable for any professional discipline to stand still, and nursing is no exception. The demands by the public, professional organisations and by nurses themselves to establish sound reasoning for the 'when, where, how and why' of nursing activities is paramount to the future of the discipline. To do this there needs to be research activity. Research is defined as 'a systematic process of investigation, the general purpose of which is to contribute to the body of knowledge that shapes and guides academic and/or practical disciplines' (Tarling and Crofts, 1998). Research is not confined to academic institutions, nor is it confined to laboratories, it is indeed part and parcel of human curiosity. It is about learning and understanding as much as possible about the world, and about seeking valid and useful information. Research is about asking questions—questions about what causes changes in behaviour, about the effectiveness of drugs to treat illness, and about the normal progression of children, to name but a few. Central to any research is that it answers a question, people will benefit from the answer and that the people who are being investigated will be treated with the greatest care and will not be harmed.

Key issues:

- Identification of different types of research

- Principles of ethical research
- Methods of protecting human subjects
- Rules for socially responsible nursing research

Types of research

Research is not just about experiments, there are many different ways in which knowledge and understanding can be gleaned: 'When we speak of research, we speak of a family of methods that share the characteristics of disciplined inquiry' (Shulman, 1990: 8). When Lee Shulman, a noted educational researcher, wrote these words he was offering new researchers two ideas. First, research is disciplined, that is, it is structured not haphazard: 'its data, arguments, and reasoning [are] capable of withstanding careful scrutiny by another member of the scientific community' (Shulman, 1990: 9). Second, Shulman was pointing out that there is no one way to do research, there are many, but they share the characteristic of being disciplined inquiry.

There are three basic types of questions that research projects can address:

(a) Descriptive

This is where a study is primarily designed to describe what is going on or what exists. Public opinion polls are descriptive when they collect details about the proportion of people who hold various opinions; for example, whether or not people agree with euthanasia.

(b) Relational

This is where a study is designed to look at the relationships between two or more issues of interest (these are called 'variables'). A public opinion poll that compares what proportion of men and women are in favour of euthanasia is essentially studying the relationship between gender and this opinion.

(c) Causal

This is where a study is designed to determine whether one or more variables—for example, a particular treatment—causes or affects one or more outcome variable. If we carried out a public opinion poll to determine whether a legal case changed the general public's opinion on euthanasia, we would be studying whether the case causes a change in the proportion of the public for and against euthanasia.

Whatever type of research question are being asked, there are numerous ways of finding the answers. For the researcher, however, it is important that the right research method is used, i.e. Randomised Controlled Trial (RCT), questionnaire, in-depth interview, or secondary analysis. Whatever the research method, there needs to be careful thought and consideration given as to what or who is being investigated. Most research that involves humans rather than, for example, a study on computer technology, needs what is termed 'ethical approval' due to the risks of physical and moral harm. In general, the only human research which does not need ethical approval, is that which uses:

- information from a public database, where collected data cannot be associated with any one individual or group of individuals
- observations of behaviour within a public gathering, that cannot be associated with any particular group or individual
- information already within the public domain, such as autobiographies, diaries or public archives.

Principles of ethical research

The historical background

The inclusion of ethical consideration in any research involving humans has only relatively recently been of international concern. Until the middle of the twentieth century, concerns about the ethics of the practice of medicine centred on therapeutic medicine as opposed to research medicine. National and international efforts to protect the rights and welfare of human subjects of research have occurred, often in response to ethical violations—situations in which researchers were found to have ignored the fundamental rights of human subjects. The most notable of these are the use of human subjects in Nazi Germany. In order to ensure the supremacy of the Aryan race, the Nazi party in Germany desired to find a secret way of sterilising large populations. Three experiments involving sterilisation were in progress when World War II ended in 1945:

- Dried plant juice was added to flour that was fed to the general population. This was supposed to sterilise women
- Intra-uterine injections of a silver nitrate solution were given to women, without their consent, during routine physical examinations
- Men standing at a counter to complete forms were exposed to large doses of X-radiation, without their knowledge.

In addition to the experiments with sterilisation, Nazi doctors were under pressure to develop a vaccine for typhus fever that could be given to the German troops. In order to develop and test such a vaccine, concentration camp prisoners were administered either vaccine or a placebo then injected with blood from prisoners who had the typhus fever.

It was not until after World War II that many of the horrors of such experiments were exposed. During the trials of war criminals at Nuremberg, fundamental ethical principles for the conduct of research involving human beings were codified into the Nuremberg Code. The Code set out ten conditions that must be met before research involving humans is ethically permissible. These concern issues, such as responsibility for gaining consent, avoiding physical and mental suffering, the need for the subject to be free to leave the research at anytime, and the correct training of the researchers. The Nuremberg Code became the first international standard for the conduct of research. Although the Code did not carry the force of law, it was the first document that advocated voluntary participation and informed consent.

Nazi Germany however, was not the only country to be involved in medical experiments with human subjects. In the United States of America in the early 1930s, a study was held to determine the natural history of untreated latent syphilis. It involved over 400 black men with syphilis. By the 1940s, when Penicillin was found to be effective in the treatment of syphilis and became available, the men in the study were neither informed nor treated with the antibiotic. The study continued until it was reported in the press in 1972. In 1963, regardless of the recommendations included in the Nuremburg Code, another infamous study was carried out. Patients who were hospitalised with various chronic debilitating diseases had live cancer cells injected. The researchers believed that the cancer cells would be rejected and stated that they had been given verbal consent by the patients, yet it transpired that the patients had not been informed that it was cancer cells which were being injected. In these actions, there was a clear violation of fundamental ethical principles.

In 1964, the World Medical Association established recommendations guiding medical staff in biomedical research involving human subjects. The Declaration of Helsinki governs research ethics and identifies four forms of research on human subjects:

- **Non-intrusive research** that does not involve direct interference with the subject. It may involve making observations or carrying out an epidemiological study from medical records, but it does not impinge in any way on the patient's mind or body

- **Intrusive research** entails direct involvement with the subject. This may be non-invasive (such as psychological enquiries) or it may involve physical invasion (such as surgical intervention)

- **Therapeutic or clinical research** involves research combined with professional care and is conducted with a view to benefiting the patients on whom it is carried out

● *Non-therapeutic or non-clinical research* is a 'purely scientific application of medical research carried out on a human being' (Declaration of Helsinki, 1989). It involves volunteers who will not, or who are unlikely to, benefit directly from the procedures, but who will provide the opportunity to further scientific knowledge. These volunteers may include people who have no connection with the illness or process under investigation, such as student volunteers or the researchers themselves.

The 18th WMA General Assembly adopted the Declaration of Helsinki in June 1964. Since then the Declaration has undergone a number of amendments, the most recent being in October 2000. The additional issues addressed in the Declaration include:

● Research with humans should be based on laboratory and animal experimentation
● An independent committee should review research protocols
● Informed consent is necessary
● Research should be conducted by medically/scientifically qualified individuals
● Risks should not exceed benefits.

Risks and benefits

The term 'risk' refers both to the probability of harm resulting from an activity and its magnitude. In other words, just how big is the risk? It is worth bearing in mind that even inactivity may be associated with some risk. However, risk does not just relate to physical harm, but also includes emotional and psychological harm. Negligible or minimal risk can be considered as equal to the probability and magnitude of physical or psychological harm that is normally encountered in one's daily life. Examples of negligible risk might include simple physiological experiments involving exercise on healthy volunteers, collecting hair and nail samples, and measuring height and weight. Clearly, in more complex studies, such as drug trials, there may be greater risks of adverse reactions.

A 'benefit' is the opposite of harm, and refers to any sort of favourable outcome to society, or to the individual. One of the difficulties which arises is that the outcome of research is never certain at the outset; therefore, there needs to be consideration of the probability of possible benefit as well as its magnitude.

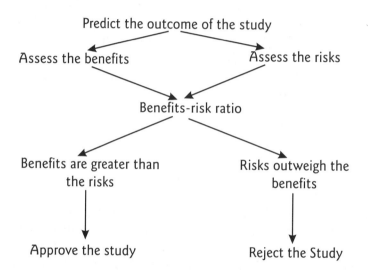

Moral theory

Deontology is the ethical theory that states that the moral rightness or wrongness of human action can be considered independent of the consequences of the action. Sometimes it is not the consequences of an action that make it right or wrong, but the principle or motivation on which the action is based that determines rightness or wrongness, i.e. in the research, is the individual treated not as a means to an end, but an end in themselves? Is the research based on beneficence, respect for patient rights, and justice without regard for the consequences? By contrast, utilitarianism is the ethical theory that encourages us to act in ways that would produce the greatest balance of good over evil. The action with the most positive consequences and the least negative physical/social consequences would be the morally preferable action, i.e. in the research, does the end justify the means? May we use a person for the good of many others and to advance knowledge even if it causes this one person a great deal of discomfort?

So far, we can see it is all about balancing the risks and benefits of the research. There is a clear responsibility to ensure that the benefits to the patient or patient group exceeds the risks/costs. The overall aim is 'to do good' and, when considering research proposals, researchers should ask themselves if they would allow a member of their own family to participate. Research that did not involve any risk or harm to anyone would be ideal, but to a large extent this would prohibit much research, particularly in health care. The role of the nurse could be said to avoid harm and, when this principle is satisfied, to assist in the provision of current or future benefits to patients (RCN Research Society, 2001). That said, there are many nursing actions which result in harm, but are balanced by more important benefits for the individual; for example, giving an injection to relieve pain, or encouraging a patient to mobilise after surgery to reduce complications. The same may be true of research where the benefits are for the majority in the future, but not necessarily to the individual at that time.

Methods of protecting human subjects

Central to any research is the protection of human participants. The key aspects are protection from physical and mental harm. The research should not cause undue suffering to the individuals and the physical and mental outcomes of the research should, on balance, benefit the research participant, and not be to their detriment. Key to protecting the participant from moral harm are the concepts of autonomy, freedom, anonymity, and informed consent. These will now be explored in more detail in relation to research.

Autonomy and Freedom

This refers to the right to make one's own decisions and, conversely, to respect the choices that others make for themselves. The researcher needs to examine:

- The relationship between autonomy and the capacity for it
- The adequacy for options
- Independence
- Aiming at the good.

The autonomous person is the author of his or her life. Individuals are believed to have self-control and are encouraged to control, as far as possible, their own destiny through making their own decisions throughout their lives. However, to be able to do this the person does need a degree of self-awareness and to be aware of what options are available. The person also needs to understand how the choices made will impact on his/her life. Autonomy is the opposite of coercion. Coercion diminishes a person's options whereas manipulation perverts the way that persons reach decisions, form preferences or adopt goals. Coercion and manipulation together will affect a person's independence/freedom, and is inconsistent with autonomy. Finally, autonomy is only of value if it is exercised in the pursuit of the good; that is, autonomy requires the availability of morally acceptable options.

Anonymity

Anonymity is where the researcher and everyone else involved in the study cannot identify who the participants are and the easiest way to achieve this is through using a questionnaire that is not coded in any way which might identify the respondent. The Data Protection Act 1998 came into force in 2000. It legislates for the control and protection of personal data. The more stringent requirements of the Act do not, however, apply to certain kinds of health care research, such as where anonymised, unlinked data is used and some types of epidemiological research, due to an 'exemption' clause. That said, the Research Governance

Framework for Health and Social Care (1998) incorporates the stipulations of the Data Protection Act and requires that, in the research setting, the appropriate use and protection of patient data are paramount. All those involved in research must be aware of their legal and ethical duties in this respect. Particular attention must be given to systems for ensuring confidentiality of personal information and to the security of these systems.

Informed consent

Informed consent is about the right to control our own destinies and to determine our own ends as far as is humanly possible; it is about the right to make choices and the right to refuse consent; it is about the right of individuals to preserve their integrity and dignity whatever physical and mental deterioration they may suffer through ill health; it is about our duty always and in all circumstances to respect each other as fellow human beings and as persons (Faulder, 1985: 2). Informed consent in research is based on the following principles:

- adequate time must be given to consider consent
- the language used must be understandable to the person
- the study must be clearly described including any side-effects or hazards
- where appropriate, alternative therapies must be described
- a statement of confidentiality must be provided
- identified persons must be available to be contacted for further questions
- a statement of voluntary participation must be obtained
- it must be made clear that consent can be withdrawn at any point in the study.

Consider the following case:

> Mrs Jamin is an 81-year-old lady with Alzheimer's disease. She is being cared for in hospital and has been asked to take part in a clinical trial to test a new drug designed to help improve memory. You were present when the researcher obtained a signed informed consent form from Mrs Jamin a few days ago. However, when you ask Mrs Jamin if she is ready to begin the study the following day she looks at you blankly and seems to have no idea what you are talking about.

One of the major issues here is the competence of Mrs Jamin to give ethically valid consent. The researcher should be contacted to discuss Mrs Jamin's participation in the trial. Mrs Jamin needs to be informed of any risks and implications of taking part in a format that is accessible, for example, written information as well as a verbal explanation. Although she may be considered to be a vulnerable research subject because of her mental status, Mrs Jamin does belong to the population the intervention is designed to assist and her participation may benefit herself and other people with Alzheimer's. However, there needs to be a careful balancing of risks and benefits. Often it is beneficial to have an advocate present for the potential participant, such as member of the family, close friend or nurse.

Generally, in research, consent should be in writing whereas when someone is consenting to healthcare that consent may be implicit. In consenting to healthcare, a patient hopes that the care will make him/her better. However, in quantitative research the focus is not on any one individual, but on the effects of an intervention on large numbers of people. Similarly, in qualitative research, the focus is not about making one individual better, but is concerned with gaining more information about that person; for example, about their beliefs, values or opinions.

It is inevitable that any individual receiving health care may feel that refusing to participate in a research study might make him/her appear ungrateful for the care given. Patients may worry that if they do not co-operate, the quality of care given may be adversely affected. Alternatively, they may go along with it simply because they believe that the doctor or nurse know best. We need to be sensitive to the fact that all individuals being given health care are vulnerable and that undue pressure, however inadvertently, may be put on patients and clients in any form of research, including nursing research. Undue pressure is not a danger solely limited to the researcher's relationship with the patient. Care staff may also be pressurised to assist or take part in research studies, believing that their job prospects may be jeopardised if they refuse.

The types of information that must be given to potential research subjects to aid informed consent, include:

- The purpose and justification for the study, which is described and explained in jargon free language
- The procedures and research interventions, including a clear distinction between research interventions and routine care and treatment
- Potential harm/risks to the individual/group, and society
- Potential benefits to the individual/group and society
- The right to withdraw at any time without routine care or treatment suffering is made explicit
- The nature of the subject's commitment
- Confidentiality pledge is stated and voluntary consent obtained
- Alternative treatments and or care that may be beneficial
- Details as to who to contact for further information and explanation if necessary

(See Polit and Hungler, 1991)

It should also be noted that consent in research is a process, and not a once-only event. Consent may need to be renegotiated over time, especially in longitudinal studies where the research may be over a number of years (for example, in studies of children's development and behaviour, or in studies of chronic disease). Researchers should also be mindful of cultural, religious, gendered and other significant differences within the research populations in the planning, conducting and reporting of their research. It should be borne in mind that the best judge of whether an investigation will cause offence may be a member of the population from which the research participants will be drawn. Apart from asking the participants themselves, there is another way in which research can be judged to be ethically sound or not, and that is through an Ethics Committee (see below).

Ethical consideration also has to be given to the actions of the researcher(s) during the steps of the research process. The following table illustrates some examples of where unethical actions may occur:

STEP	UNETHICAL ACTIONS
Defining purpose of study	Waste of resources (research not important). Misleading or fraudulent. Unnecessary research for financial/ personal gain.
Literature search	Biassed search and review. Conflicting evidence ignored. Quoting out of context. Plagiarism.
Data Collection	Intentionally using data collection methods to get intended/biassed data. Bribing for data. Falsifying/fabricating data.
Data Analysis	Ignoring contradictory data. Manipulating data to achieve intended/biassed findings. Intentional loss/destruction of data.
Conclusions/ recommendations	Intentionally misleading or false conclusions and or recommendations. Intentional withholding of conclusions and recommendations.

STEP	UNETHICAL ACTIONS
Communicating/ publishing	Withholding communicating or publishing. Communicating or publishing selected parts only for unacceptable reasons Breaking confidentiality.

Rules for socially responsible research

Ethics committees

Due to the need for ethical consideration of research involving humans, and that most research in the NHS accesses vulnerable people, local research committees (LRECS) have been set up. In the UK, these committees are only concerned with research and are not committees that can be called upon when one has an ethical dilemma in practice.

In 1968, the Department of Health recommended that hospitals should operate ethics committees, but it was not until 1984 that the Royal College of Physicians produced guidelines and it was 1990 before such committees were formally termed LRECs. Their brief was to 'maintain ethical standards of practice in research, to protect subjects of research from harm, to preserve subjects' rights and to provide reassurance to the public that this is being done (COREC, 2004). LRECs not only safeguard the research subjects, they also safeguard the researchers themselves. In 1997, a system of Multi-centre Research Ethics Committees (MRECs) was set up. An MREC is an advisory body providing independent advice on the science and general ethics of multi-centre proposals. A multi-centre proposal is one where subjects are recruited from five or more districts.

Any nurse taking part in a research project in whatever capacity should be told whether LREC consent was obtained as this indicates that any ethical issues have been addressed. Examples of research that will need ethical approval, include:

- Clinical trials involving testing new drugs on patients and clients
- Clinical trials involving testing new drugs on healthy volunteers
- Asking patients to complete a questionnaire
- Interviewing patients or clients
- Taking a blood sample from a patient or client
- Taking a blood sample from a healthy volunteer
- Asking hospital or care staff to complete a questionnaire
- Interviewing staff
- Research carried out as part of an academic programme
- Research on specimens and tissues/organs removed during surgery or other procedure
- Research involving patient/client medical notes (where the patient is not present)
- Research carried out by another organisation on hospital/care premises
- Observational studies.

(Tarling and Crofts, 1998)

The role of the nurse in research

The nurse may be involved in research in a variety of ways:

- Helping write the research
- Carrying out the research
- Caring for the patients who are research participants
- Supporting a patient who has been approached to take part in a research study
- Reading the research to base practice on.

Although the role of the nurse will be different in each situation, the ethical principles already discussed will apply equally. The nurse must also:

- be aware of potential bias
- always seek to do the best research possible
- seek advice on ethical issues.

An Exercise

Mr B is a patient on a medical ward. He is involved in a research project, which is testing the efficacy of a new drug. The research is in the form of a randomised control trial and as the nurse who is caring for Mr B, you do not know if he is receiving the trial drug or the conventional drug treatment. In conversation with you, Mr B admits that he really does not understand the study and his part in it. He is unsure if he wants to continue, but is very concerned that his medical treatment will be affected if he asks to leave the study.

Questions:

1.   Has the participant given his/her consent?

2.   Has the participant been coerced in any way?

3.   Has information about the true nature of the research been withheld?

4.   Has the participant been deceived in any way?

5.   Has the participant been made to feel uncomfortable or humiliated?

6.   Has his/her rights of self-determination been violated?

7.   Has the participant been exposed to unnecessary physical or mental stress?

8. Has his/her privacy been violated?

9. Have benefits been withheld?

10. Has the participant been treated fairly, with respect and consideration?

In our example, Mr B has to have the freedom to leave the study at any time without fear of repercussions and without coercion. This can be difficult where there is a power difference between the researcher and the researched, or where there has been some form of inducement to participate. Patients not uncommonly feel that their care may be compromised if they withdraw. If their freedom to withdraw has not been fully explained, then this in itself is a form of manipulation and coercion.

In Mr B's study anonymity has not been achieved. Although he is not aware of which group (experimental/control) he is in, the researcher would be able to identify him through a coding system. However, what Mr B should expect is the fundamental right of confidentiality. On completion of the study, there should be no one outside the research team who could identify the respondents. This requires meticulous attention to detail, in that any possible identifying information about the respondents must be removed.

With reference to Mr B, it is debatable whether informed consent was obtained. Either the information given was insufficient or at the wrong level. In addition, it appears that his voluntariness was violated. Mr B was not truly participating of his own free will and felt coerced into taking part. He has informed you that he is worried about his future care should he withdraw. In this case, the researchers need to have further discussions with him. The nurse thereby acts as his advocate.

Conclusion

To conclude, consider the following perspectives for assessing ethical acceptability. From the utilitarian perspective, the good of a research project is determined by the expected consequences of its results in terms of 'the greatest good for the greatest number'. Note that, sometimes, this can seem to allow that the end justifies the means. Also, researchers may have a different idea about the value of various consequences. From the deontological perspective, there are absolute imperatives that place moral restrictions on research activities. For example, the deontologist might insist that deception in experiments is never justified no matter what the positive contributions of knowledge. Note that some deontologists are more flexible, making a distinction between harm and wrong (harms can be compensated for but wrongs cannot). The main principles of ethical research are respect for persons, which grounds the moral requirements of informed consent, autonomy, privacy, confidentiality; and non-maleficence, and beneficence, which ground the duties not to inflict harm, to promote good, to minimise risk and to maximise benefit; and justice, which grounds the requirement to undertake research fairly. The main methods of protecting human research participants are:

- Gain informed consent
- Gain ethics approval from the relevant ethics committee
- Abide by rules for socially responsible nursing research
- Distinguish between science and advocacy
- Do not search the data in support of your own views
- Be aware of potential bias
- Represent the literature fairly
- Always seek to do the best research possible
- Acknowledge your sources
- Seek advice on ethical issues.

References

COREC (2004) Central Office for Research Ethics Committees. www.corec.org.uk

Data Protection Act (1991) HMSO, London

Declaration of Helsinki (1989) Recommendations guiding physicians. In: *Biomedical Research Involving Human Subjects.* World Medical Association

Department of Health (2001) *Research Governance Framework for Health And Social Care.* Department of Health, London

Faulder C (1985)*Whose Body is it? The Troublesome Issue of Consent.* Virago Press, London UK

Polit DF, Hungler BP (1991) *Nursing Research: Principles and Methods*, 4th edn. Lippencott, London

RCN Research Society (2001) Royal College of Nursing Research and Development Co-ordination Centre.

Shulman LS (1990) *Paradigms and Programs: Research in Teaching and Learning.* Macmillan, USA

Tarling M, Crofts L (1998) *The Essential Researcher's Handbook for Nurses and Healthcare Professionals.* Bailliere Tindall, London

Further reading

Tingle J, Cribb A (2002) *Nursing Law and Ethics*, 2nd edn. Blackwell Publishing, London

Thompson IE, Melia KM, Boyd KM (2002) *Nursing Ethics.* Churchill Livingstone, London

Websites

www.wma.net/L/policy/17-c

www.corec.org.uk

www.doh.gov.uk/research

Main Codes for Ethical Decision-Making

Nuremburg Code
Declaration of Helsinki
American Nurses Association Code of Ethics
Code of Professional Conduct (NMC 2002)

8

CULTURAL DIVERSITY

K Fritz

Introduction

'For whites, race is like a sauce—we can put on as little or as much of it as we desire.
For blacks, race is like a marinade—it permeates everything'

(Alcorn, 2000)

In a small hospital near the coast, a first generation woman from India was admitted to a surgical ward. She was not able to speak fluent English and did not ask for much attention from the nurses. Her young family members visited her every evening. In order to gain informed consent to a gynaecological operation, the surgeon asked the 10-year-old grandson to interpret for him. The next day another Asian woman was admitted, so the staff decided to put her into the bed next to the woman from India, so that they could chat and keep each other company. However, the second woman was from Pakistan, visiting her English grandchildren. She was not from the same ethnic group, did not speak the same language, did not share the same religious beliefs and, by virtue of her nationality, considered Indian people to be her political 'enemies'.

What are the ethical issues within this scenario? How might the nursing staff have dealt with these situations more effectively? What knowledge base might they have needed? What skills are important? In this chapter, we look at what underpins the nurse's role within a context of cultural diversity. While we focus on cultural diversity, many of the same principles apply to other types of diversity, e.g.

age, gender, disability, religion, and lifestyle. There are ethical, legal, professional and even personal grounds for embracing equality within diversity and these will be addressed briefly. In order to be able to celebrate diversity, it is important to begin with an awareness of one's own culture and then to move from that self-awareness to develop a positive regard for others. We will address common words used within cultural diversity and briefly examine the theoretical foundations, the importance of attitudes and the necessary skills. The interrelationship between culture and health will be looked at from three perspectives—expectations, explanations and equity. There are exercises, case studies and reflection points in order to help you to get the most out of this chapter.

Key issues

- Cultural self-awareness: an exercise
- Why nurses need to address this issue: the foundations
- Common terminology
- Knowledge base: what nurses need to know
- The importance of attitudes: prejudice and discrimination
- Helpful skills to develop: communication and interpersonal relationship skills
- The interaction between culture and health.

Learning outcomes:

- To understand your own values and attitudes and how these may affect others
- To identify skills that are appropriate to cultural diversity and health
- To explore relevant areas of knowledge, including prejudice and discrimination
- To recognise the relationship between culture and health

- To appreciate the ethical issues related to cultural diversity.

Your culture

Each of us brings our own values and beliefs to our experiences with people from different backgrounds. It is important to be aware of what we value and what we feel about practices that differ from ours and to know why. In the past, a 'colour-blind' approach (treating everyone the same) was adopted; this resulted in a failure to recognise the ways in which people's needs are individual. A person who believes s/he is 'colour blind' and 'treats everyone the same' is failing to treat people appropriately as individuals and, rather than challenging racism, is helping to perpetuate it. Inequity is often based on stereotyping, prejudice and racism. You have a culture of your own. It may surprise you to consider this, as you may have always thought that you are the 'norm'. In order to understand more about your culture, experience and values, do the following exercise:

An exercise: My culture and values

Step 1

1. In the centre of a blank piece of paper, write your name;

2. Underneath write your ethnic group, religion, age group, community;

3. In one corner, write the experiences you have had with people from ethnic groups, religions, age groups or communities different from your own;

4. In the second corner, name one thing about your ethnic group, religion, age group or community that you find embarrassing or wish you could change;

5. In the third corner, write two values from your child-hood that relate to your own 'culture'. Who taught you these values? Do these values influence you today? How? If not, why not?

6. In the fourth corner, draw a symbol or identify an item that typifies your 'culture' or a major aspect of it (for example, a mobile phone).

Step 2

1. Discuss your results with a friend or classmate:
    - Are your backgrounds and values similar? Why?
    - Are your backgrounds and values different? Why?

2. Discuss with your colleague your feelings about work-ing with people who have backgrounds and values dif-ferent from yours.

3. Share your knowledge and views of the values of people from other cultures.

[Adapted from Spradley BW, Allender JA (1996); Chitty KK (1997); Clark MJ (1996); In: Andrews and Boyle P (1999) *Transcultural Concepts in Nursing Care*, 3rd edn: 447; and Yvie Holder (2001) 'Who am I?' quiz.]

Reflection point

Imagine entering hospital in a place where your ethnic group is a minority. What would be important for you in terms of:

- diet
- religious practices
- privacy, modesty
- visitors.

Most people have seen or experienced racism. Have you? What was your experience? What were your feelings? How might you behave differently because of that experience? What might it be like to experience racism on a daily basis?

The historical context

An historical look at Britain shows how greatly the British Empire has influenced the ethnic make-up of Britain today. In the 1950s, labourers were brought from various Commonwealth countries in order to staff industries, such as the textile mills. A shipload of Jamaican nurses came to England to staff the first NHS hospitals in 1948. Currently, nurses and other medical professions are being recruited internationally. Through immigration (and each country's immigrants are another country's emigrants), Britain has become a community of communities; everyone belongs to more than one community and these overlap and influence each other. While it is impossible to know every aspect of all the subcultures, it may be helpful to know some key aspects of the major cultural groups in order to be able to nurse with knowledge. Try answering the quiz below:

1. Name at least seven cultural groups or subcultures in or near where you work or live.

2. What are the five 'k's that are important in Sikhism?

3. What are the five pillars of Islam?

4. What are the five divisions of the caste system?

5. What do you know about the main dietary considerations for the following groups?
   - Hindus
   - Jews
   - Rastafarians
   - Muslims
   - Seventh Day Adventists

- Roman Catholics
- Mormons

6. What language do Muslims speak?

7. Name three religions of China;

8. Name some of the Caribbean islands;

9. What difficulties do the English terms 'please' and 'thank you' pose for intercultural communication?

10. What cultural considerations might others need to know about the British?

11. Write down any forms of address that you know from different languages;

12. Write down some lifestyle conventions of different cultural groups that might be important for interaction.

[Adapted from Chouhan 2000 (suggested answers are at the end of the chapter)]

How culture can affect health

Cultural beliefs and values, traditions and customs can affect both individual and societal health, with either a positive or a negative effect. Using three 'Es', we can summarise some ways in which this happens.

Explanations

The explanations of what health is and what causes disease can affect the cures and solutions which people seek. Many cultures believe that illness and disability are caused by evil spirits or bewitching. Some explanations, for example in Islam, are based on the humoural theory (the body has four fluids—yellow bile, blood, phlegm, black bile—

which must remain in balance). Where there is an imbalance, the type is diagnosed by traditional practitioners and hot or cold foods must be avoided in an effort to restore the balance. The Chinese explanation on the balance of Yin and Yang is similar and foods, again classified as hot or cold, are part of the treatment. The western system of medicine is based on the biomedical model, stemming from Cartesian theory separating mind and body. The body is seen as a machine, so parts can be replaced.

Expectations

Health and disease may be measured differently in each culture. The common illnesses, life expectancy, and common causes of death, will influence people's behaviour. In Glasgow, 12% of people interviewed in a study had chronic bronchitis, so they considered this to be a normal condition, rather than something to treat and cure. For those in minority groups, Kleinman (1980) identified three overlapping sectors of health care:

- popular sector: where illness is first realised and treated; this may be within the family
- folk sector: where healing is derived from sacred and/or secular sources, e.g. from healers who share the cultural values and beliefs
- dominant views and systems in the society: here, the biomedical model and the NHS.

There may sometimes be conflict between the treatments offered by carers in these sectors, which might lead to confusion or non-compliance.

Equity

Equity means equal, fair or impartial treatment, rather than uniformity. In order to treat people equally as individuals, it may be necessary to treat them differently. Areas where equity is important, include access to health care, education, jobs, justice and access to treatment that is culturally appropriate. The influence of socio-economic factors should not be underestimated. In Britain, 70% of ethnic minorities live in the 88 most deprived local authority wards. This limits the type of services available to them.

Foundational backgrounds

Legislation

The rights in the European Convention on Human Rights became domestic law in October 2000, when the Human Rights Act came into force. These directives say that everyone, individually and in common with others, has the right to be respected for, and to express, his values and cultural traditions in so far as these are not contrary to the requirements of human dignity, human rights and fundamental freedoms. That right includes:

- the freedom to engage in cultural activity, whether in public or in private, and more particularly to speak the language of one's choice
- the entitlement to identify with the cultural communities of one's choice and to maintain relations with them (this implies freedom to alter such choice or not to identify with any cultural community)
- the right to discover the whole range of cultures, which together constitute the common heritage of humanity
- the right to knowledge of human rights and to participate in establishing a culture governed by human rights.

The Race Relations Act of 1976 made direct and indirect discrimination and victimisation unlawful in areas such as employment, education, housing, facilities and services. The Race Relations Amendment Act of 2000 outlaws race discrimination and introduces a new and enforceable duty on public bodies (including health and education—the NHS and universities) to promote racial equality. The RRAA imposes a general duty with three strands: to eliminate unlawful racial discrimination, to promote equality of opportunity, and to promote good race relations between people of different racial groups. Specific duties support the general duty by calling on each organisation to prepare a race equality scheme or policy and to monitor and publish performance by ethnic groups in relation to the key functions (e.g. employment) of the organisation.

Other relevant legislation includes:

- Sex Discrimination Act 1975
- Disability Discrimination Act 1995
- Public Order Act 1986

Government initiatives

Various government initiatives address diversity and inclusion issues:

- Saving Lives—Our Healthier Nation (1999: this promotes the setting of local targets to decrease health inequalities)
- The Vital Connection: An Equalities Framework for the NHS (Nov 1999)
- 1999 Health Survey for England (final results published January 2001)
- Commission on the Future of Multiethnic Britain (The Parekh Report, October 2000)
- European Union Race and Employment Directives (this requires member states to introduce legislation to outlaw unfair discrimination on the basis of race, sexual orientation, religion or belief, disability or age)
- Race Equality in Public Services (February 2001)
- Improving Working Lives (2001: a human resources model of good practice)

Professional imperatives

The Nursing and Midwifery Council, the statutory professional body which governs nursing has published guidelines in the NMC Professional Code of Conduct (2002); item 2 is particularly relevant:

2.   As a registered nurse or midwife, you must respect the patient or client as an individual:

>   2. 2   you are personally accountable for ensuring that you promote and protect the interests and dignity of patients and clients, irrespective of *gender, age, race, ability, sexuality, economic status, lifestyle, culture and religious or political beliefs.*

The Royal Collage of Nursing (RCN) represents nurses and nursing, endeavouring to promote excellence in practice and to shape health policies. A Diversity Group was established in 2002 to address diversity and equity issues.

Recurrent problems

Case study one

In a predominantly white area, a black African Caribbean mental health nurse, who speaks English well but with an accent, is passed over for promotion in favour of a white female nurse who has less time in the organisation. This is in spite of the fact that he has done additional training, worked on project groups and taken more than his share of unsocial hours. He is angry and wishes to take the matter further with his managers.

- What support might he find on which to base his complaint?

Case study two

A 78-year-old Irish Catholic man refused to let a black student nurse do his personal hygiene and care. He wanted to have someone else who was white and he didn't mind whether the carer was female or male.

- What might be at the root of his request?

- What does this reveal about the patient?
- What ought the nurse manager do about this?

Case study three

A devout Muslim woman was admitted to a medical ward in hospital. She was there for four days, but there was no Halal diet available so she ate only toast for four days. The student nurse was the only staff member who expressed concern about this poor diet. She offered to ask the family to bring in food, but the patient refused as she hoped to be discharged the next day.

- What should have prevented this problem?

Case study four

A patient who was on a life support machine was declared dead; his relatives were asked about the donation of his organs. They agreed to that on condition that these be given only to a white recipient.

- What are the ethical issues here?
- What should the hospital staff do?

Combatting recurrent problems

What is required of nurses to combat the following recurrent problems?

Attitudes

Our attitudes are revealed in our behaviour. These are so deep-rooted that sometimes we must change our behaviour so that our attitudes might follow. This is the reason that legislation is important; it requires certain behavioural standards, with or without the right attitudes. Nurses come into contact with people from all backgrounds, all cultures, all traditions. An open-minded and non-judgmental attitude is an essential frame of mind to cultivate, but, beyond that, positive regard and actively seeking to understand others can add a further dimension to the role and increase job satisfaction. The advocacy and empowering roles of nurses are enhanced through a more thorough familiarity with clients and colleagues from other cultures. It is important to avoid stereotypes, which are based on ignorance, assumption, historical ideas and an unwillingness to change. The stereotype of an English person as someone who eats fish and chips and stops at 4:00 pm for tea is clearly out-dated, but may still be held as true in some areas of the world. Stereotypes are a barrier to real communication.

Skills

There have been two approaches to the debate on how best to teach issues related to cultural diversity. The first has been an emphasis on developing the basic knowledge related to major cultures; this carries with it the danger of stereotyping people. For example, knowing that a man is a Hindu might encourage the nurse to make assumptions about him without checking these out. This does not promote holistic and individualised care. The second approach has been to move away from giving student nurses a thorough knowledge about the main cultural groups. Instead, the emphasis has been on addressing the attitudes which lead to racism, prejudice and discrimination. The problem with this approach is that attitudes may not change easily and behavioural changes may not follow. The compromise position recommended by Gerrish, Husband and Mackenzie (1996) is that both need to be done and that therein lies the skill. At the heart of this approach is good communication skills—listening, questioning, clarifying, reflecting, building bridges. In the example above, knowing some of the basic tenets of the Hindu faith might prepare the nurse to ask relevant and insightful questions and to listen in a receptive way to the needs of the client. Communication skills should also help you to challenge prejudice and discrimination when you come across them.

Commonalities

In recognising and appreciating diversity, it is also important to highlight similarities and celebrate commonalities. For example, the Golden Rule is found in many religions:

- Hinduism: This is the sum of duty: do naught to others which if done to thee would cause pain (The Mahabharata)
- Buddhism: Hurt not others with that which pains yourself (Udana-Varga)
- Judaism: What is hateful to you, do not to your fellow men. That is the entire law; all the rest is commentary (The Talmud)
- Zoroastrianism: That nature only is good when it shall not do unto another whatever is not good for its own self (Dadistan-I-Dinik)
- Islam: No one of you is a believer until he desires for his brother that which he desires for himself (Hadith)
- Baha'i Faith: He should not wish for others that which he doth not wish for himself, nor promise that which he doth not fulfil (Gleanings)
- Christianity: Do unto others that which you would have others do unto you (Bible)

Knowledge

In order to develop as nurses, we must build upon factual knowledge rather than on supposition, assumption and stereotypes. One of the building blocks to increasing your knowledge about diversity is to understand the language. However, terms do change and go in and out of fashion, so these need to be updated throughout your nursing career.

An exercise

Match the following terms with their definitions:

1	That complex whole which includes knowledge, beliefs, art, morals, law, custom, and other capabilities which forms the basis for an individual's identity.	a	positive action
2	The tendency to view the beliefs, assumptions, norms and values of one's own culture as the norm against which to judge another culture with different values and assumption. It assumes that one's own cultural patterns are the 'natural' and best way of acting.	b	racism
3	Making broad generalisations about particular groups of people and expecting all members of that group to think and behave identically.	c	multicultur- alism
4	Literally, pre-judging people in a negative way according to pre-conceived ideas about them.	d	culture
5	the collective failure of an organisation to provide an appropriate and professional service to people because of their colour, culture or ethnic origin.	e	stereotyping
6	the belief that many different cultures should be encouraged and allowed to flourish in society and that services and facilities, such as health, education, the arts, etc., should be delivered in a way that embodies and promotes this belief.	f	institutional racism
7	treating people more favourably on the grounds of race, nationality, religion, gender, etc (The Race Relations Act makes this illegal in the UK)	g	prejudice
8	set of attitudes and behaviour towards another racial or ethnic group based on the belief that natural differences in physical characteristics (such a skin colour, hair type, face shape, etc) correspond directly to differences in personality and ability	h	positive discrimination
9	offering special help to people who are disadvantaged because of prejudice, stereotyping and discrimination, in order that they may take full and equal advantage of opportunities in jobs, education, training, services, etc.	i	ethnicity

10	a sense of cultural and historical identity based on belonging by birth to a distinctive cultural group.	j	ethnocentrism

[Adapted from Cashmore and Ellis (1997) Dictionary of Race and Ethnic Relations, 4th ed. Answers are provided at the end of the chapter.]

Summary

As a nurse you will be in a unique position to benefit mutually through contact with clients and colleagues from culturally diverse backgrounds. In order to behave ethically, you need to have a high and continually developing degree of self-awareness. It is important to understand your own values and attitudes and how these may affect others, as well as how their values and attitudes affect you. You must continually assess your attitudes and your communication skills in order to develop those that are appropriate to cultural diversity and health. As society and cultures change and develop, you need to explore areas of knowledge that are relevant to your practice and your environment. Beware of prejudice and discrimination, whether individual or institutional. These can adversely affect health. It is important to appreciate the ethical issues inherent in appropriately treating individuals within their cultural contexts.

References

Alcorn R (2000) *Dominion*. Multnomah Publishers Inc, USA

Andrews M, Boyle J (1999) *Transcultural Concepts in Nursing Care*. Lippincott, Philadelphia

Cashmore E, Cashmore E (1997) *Dictionary of Race and Ethnic Relations*, 4th edn. Routledge, London

Chouhan K (2000) Cultural Knowledge Quiz. Unpublished quiz used at DeMontfort University, Leicester.

Gerrish K, Husband C, Mackenzie J (1996) *Nursing for a Multi-ethnic Society*. Open University Press, Buckingham

Holder Y (2001) Who am I? Unpublished quiz used at University of York

KleinmanA (1980) *Patients and Healers in the Context of Culture*. University of California Press, Berkeley

Further reading

Ahmad W, ed (1996) *'Race' and Health in Contemporary Britain*. Open University Press, Buckingham

Atkins K, Rollings J (1993) *Community Care in a Multi-racial Britain: A Critical Review of the Literature*. HMSO, London

Black J (1989) *Child Health in a Multicultural Society*. British Medical Journal, London

Dobson S (1991) *Transcultural Nursing*. Scutari Press, London

Fatchett A (1995) *Childhood to Adolescence*. Balliere Tindall, London

Helman C (1990) *Culture, Health and Illness*. Wright, London

Jogee M. Lal S (1999) *Religions and Cultures: Guide to Beliefs and Customs for Health Staff and Social Care Services*. Religions and Culture Publications, Edinburgh

Karmi G (1996) *The Ethnic Health Handbook: A Factfile for Health Care Professionals*. Blackwell Scientific, Oxford

Karseras P, Hopkins E (1987) *British Asians Health in the Community*. John Wiley and Sons, Chichester

Mares P, Henley A (1985) *Health Care in Multicultural Britain*. Health Education Council/National Extension College, Cambridge

McAvoy B, Donaldson L, eds (1990) *Health Care for Asians*. Oxford University Press, Oxford

McNaught A (1987) *Heath Action and Ethnic Minorities*. Bedford Square Press, London

Mir G, Nocon A, Ahman W, Jones L (2000) *Learning Difficulties and Ethnicity—Report to the Department of Health*. HMSO, London

Neuberger J (1994) *Caring for Dying People of Different Faiths*, 2nd edn. Mosby, London

Payer L (1990) *Medicine and Culture, Notions of Health and Sickness in Britain, the US, France and West Germany*. Victor Gollancz, London

Robinson L (1998) *'Race', Communication and the Caring Professions*. Open University Press, Buckingham

Schott J, Henley A (1997) *Culture, Religion and Childbearing in a multiracial Society*. Butterworth Heineman, Oxford

Smaje C (1995) *Health 'Race' and Ethnicity, Making Sense of the Evidence*. King's Fund Institute, London

Web sites

Commission for Racial Equality: http://www.cre.gov.uk

National Statistics: http://www.statstics.gov.uk

The 1990 Trust http://www.blink.org.uk

Transcultural Nursing Society:
http://www.trans_Hlt512403660_Hlst512403661c_Hlt512403
700BM_1_BM_2_uBM_3_lturalnursing.org

Hospital/health care Chaplaincy: http://212.36.148.211/nhscsc/
recommendbookmulticultural.html

Equality Challenge Unit, 3rd Floor, Tavistock Place, London
WC1H 9RA

A question of culture: answers

1.   Name at least seven cultural groups or subcultures in or near where you work or live.

Answer might include: Travellers; Muslim; Chinese; Japanese; Jewish; Irish; European groups; subcultures, such as rural, student, hospital.

2.   What are the five 'k's in relation to Sikhism?

Answer: Kara (steel bangle); kirpan (symbolic daggar); kesh (uncut hair); kaccha (symbolic undershorts worn by men); kangha (comb).

3.   *What are the five pillars of Islam?*

Answer: Haj (trip to Mecca); prayer five times a day (salah); alms (zakat); fasting for a month every year (saum); shahadah (profession of faith—Allah is the one true God and Mohammad is his prophet).

4.   *What are the five divisions of the caste system?*

Answer: Brahman—priests; kshatriya—warriors; vaisyas—merchants and business people; shedra—workers; harijan—untouchables (this has been outlawed in India but vestiges remain).

5.   *What do you know about the main dietary considerations for the following groups?*

Answer:

- Hindus: may depend upon caste—no beef; no alcohol; higher castes are usually vegetarian
- Jews: kosher food; no pork; no shellfish; milk and meat separate for orthodox Jews
- Rastafarians: vegetarians; no pork; no fruits of the vine (alcohol)
- Muslims: no pork; no alcohol; Halal meat (sacrificed in a ritual way)
- Seventh Day Adventists: some eat no meat; others no pork; no alcohol
- Roman Catholics: fish on Friday
- Mormons: no caffeine; no alcohol

6.   *What language do Muslims speak?*

Answer: Many, depending on their nationality.

7. Name three religions of China.

Answer might include: Taoism; Buddhism; Zen; Confucianism; Christianity.

8. Name some of the Caribbean islands.

Answer might include: Jamaica; Tobago; Trinidad; St Kit; St Nevis; Cuba.

9. What difficulties do the English terms 'please' and 'thank you' pose for intercultural communication?

Answer: Sometimes these are used synonymously; meanings may be unclear; there may be no equivalents; these are often built into phrasing.

10. What cultural considerations might others need to know about the British?

Answer might include: work ethic; body language; eye contact; modesty; queuing; emotions; rich historical background; sense of humour and irony; youth/drink culture; football allegiance.

11. Write down any forms of address that you know from different languages.

Answer might include: Salaam alekum; namaste; might include gestures of greeting or welcome.

12. *Write down some lifestyle conventions of different cultural groups that might be important for interaction.*

Answer might include: religious beliefs and values (e.g. prayers); dietary needs; beliefs and rituals related to dying and death and other life events; language and communications including gestures; attitudes towards children; importance of families; hospitality; customs; traditions.

Answers to the final Exercise: 1d; 2j; 3e; 4g; 5f; 6c; 7h; 8b; 9a; 10i

9

RESOURCE ALLOCATION

C Clarke

Introduction

How to ration health care resources is one of the most debated and contentious issues currently facing the National Health Service (New and Grand, 1996). There are many expensive things that medicine can do, but the question ethics asks is, 'should we do them?' (Singer, 1994). The main aim of this chapter is to identify the ethical issues related to the just distribution of these limited health care resources. It is hoped that by the end of this chapter, you will have begun to critically reflect on the some of the key ethical issues and difficulties such decisions pose.

Advances in medical science and technology, escalating costs, the limited availability of certain health care resources, such as organs for transplantation, time or the personnel to deliver the care, together with an increasing number of older people, has created a gap between supply and demand. In addition, public expectations about what health care can and should offer continue to rise. Some form of rationing and patient selection appears inevitable, but this can be achieved in a number of different ways and it is this debate that has created considerable public and political controversy and media interest. It is important to note, however, that rationing has always been present within the National Health Service, although it is not the case that the public perceived this to be the case (New and Grand, 1996). Rationing was therefore implicit in nature and patients were often told they did not need treatment rather than that treatment was unavailable because of limited resources (Hunter, 1997). The medical profession, who had considerable influence, controlled the rationing and distribution of the available, sometimes limited, resources. Attempts have now been made to prioritise and re-allocate resources in a more systematic and rational manner according to agreed systems or criteria. This has made the issue of rationing explicit and open to debate.

Learning outcomes

- Define justice and identify some possible approaches
- Define the problem of resource allocation at a macro and micro level
- Discuss ways to decide what is on the menu
- Discuss the criterion to be used to decide who is chosen for treatment
- Discuss who should make the relevant decisions.

Justice, equity, efficiency and effectiveness

Justice as a moral principle is about justice as fairness, rather than justice as retribution; it is defined as 'fair, equitable and appropriate distribution in society (Beachamp and Childress, 1994: 237). An injustice involves a wrongful act or omission that denies an individual benefits to which he/she has a right, or fails to distribute burdens or benefits fairly. Endeavouring to decide what counts as a 'right' or a legitimate claim in health care poses many problems. Some possible approaches, called 'principles of justice', are:

- To each person an equal share
- To each person a share according to effort
- To each person a share according to contribution
- To each person a share according to merit
- To each person a share according to free market exchanges.

(Beauchamp and Childress, 1994)

No single principle of justice is capable of addressing all the problems, and conflicts among them create a serious priority problem. Common to all theories of justice is a 'decent minimum' requirement rather than optimum care. Health care today is largely based on a utilitarian theory of justice: i.e. that all social goods and services should be distributed so as to maximise utility. A criticism of this theory of distribution is that, in pursuit of maximising, insufficient weight is given to the rights of the individual to fairness and equality.

However, it is important to consider what 'equality' in health care actually requires: equal in relation to what, over what period of time and with respect to what criteria? For example, does it mean equal access, an equal chance or opportunity to receive health care resources or treatment, or equal respect in relation to the resource? It is unrealistic to imagine that some life-sustaining treatment, for example, heart transplantation, can be provided for everyone based on medical need or demand. If a right to equal treatment exists and requires that, if treatment be provided to some then it must be provided to all, the overall expenditure on health would reach huge proportions and this might result in treatments being provided to none because limited resources would not enable the treatment to be available to everyone. This would result in the standards of health care being lowered and also have an impact on the advancement of certain treatments at an experimental stage (Fried, 1983). Therefore, some inequalities in the treatment available might be morally justified, provided the decision to treat some rather than all was not based on morally irrelevant traits, such as race or gender.

Also, allocating resources to maximise benefit has resulted in restricting services to those that are effective and efficient. An effective treatment is defined as one that produces a desirable health outcome, for example, recovery from an operation. An efficient treatment is one where output is maximised from a given input of resources (see Williams, 2001). Making a judgement about the effectiveness and efficiency of various health care treatments is complex and creates considerable difficulties in practice.

The effectiveness or outcome of treatment is rarely certain and often disputed, and requires the collection of precise and accurate clinical data regarding the outcome of various treatment options. It is also possible for a treatment to be effective, but not efficient. Restricting treatment to those that are effective and efficient can also create conflict between the needs of the individual and society as a whole. Harris (1996) argues that the drive to maximise the benefit of health care resources has resulted in choosing the patient with the best prognosis, which can result in discrimination and the unequal treatment of individuals. Efficiency, which according to Culyer (1997) is what maximising is about, sometimes needs to be tempered by considerations of equity in both process and outcome. But, in situations where these principles conflict, how does one weigh one against another?

The cost-effectiveness of treatment also needs to be considered. Williams (1989) argues that:

> '...to ignore costs is unethical because it means ignoring avoidable death and suffering. People who refuse to count the costs of their actions are not behaving ethically, they are behaving fanatically and fanaticism has no place in the practice of medicine.'

Cost effectiveness in purely financial terms is an important consideration, but not the only issue as other costs need to be taken into account, such as how acceptable the treatment is to the patient and what side-effects might result from treatment.

Case Study

A patient is admitted to an ICU with a life-threatening physiological event and without immediate intervention will almost certainly die. However, the outcome of treatment is uncertain and the mortality rate amongst patients with this severity of illness is high. It actually costs 2–3 times more to die on an intensive care unit than it does to survive (Mostafa, 1995). The provision of intensive care facilities involves a substantial cost for a small number of patients. It costs 3–5 times more than a bed on a general ward. There-fore, a large proportion of the hospital budget is spent on individuals with limited chance of benefit in terms of survival.

- Should life-sustaining treatment always take priority over life-enhancing treatment?
- What about preventive treatment and mental health?
- Is spending large amounts of limited resources on individuals with little prospect of recovery cost-effective and justified?

Problem of distributive justice only occur when there is a shortage of goods within society. Limited resources create competition and the need to establish priorities and make choices at all levels. Within the health care system competition for resources occurs at two levels. At the macro-level, the main question is, What should be rationed? At the micro-level, it is, How should rationing be conducted between individuals competing for the same scarce resource (see New and Grand, 1996)?

Macro-allocation

In order to prioritise and maximise the benefit of health care expenditure, it is necessary to find a way of measuring benefit or heath gain (Williams, 2001). Traditionally, the measure used was survival rates or life-years gained, but factors other than survival count. For example, some procedures, such as total hip replacements, have little effect on life expectancy but do improve quality of life by reducing pain and disability. QALYs (Quality Adjusted Life Years) work by measuring and comparing the outcomes of different health care interventions and treatments in terms of both quality and length of life. According to Williams (1985):

'The essence of a QALY is that it takes a year of healthy life expectancy to be worth one, but regards a year of

unhealthy life expectancy to be worth less than one. The precise value is lower the worse the quality of life of the unhealthy person. If being dead is worth zero it is, in principle, possible for a QALY to be negative, the quality of someone's life to be judged worse than death.'

The general idea is that a beneficial health care activity is one that generates a positive number of QALYs and that an efficient health care activity is one where the cost per QALY is as low as can be. A high priority health care activity is one where the cost per QALY is low, and a low priority activity is one where the cost per QALY is high. The main aim of the QALY approach to health care is to ensure that as much benefit as possible is obtained from resources devoted to health care. Comparisons can be made between a QALY approach and a utilitarian approach to resource allocations, as both act so as to maximise aggregate benefit. Benefit is measured in terms of the effect of treatment on life expectancy adjusted for the quality of life.

The use of the QALY, as with a utilitarian approach, requires the calculation of the utility of actions. However, it is impossible to predict with absolute certainty the benefit or outcome of some treatments in terms of future life expectancy or quality of life. Sometimes, this can only be calculated after a trial period of treatment and can only ever be a judgment of probability not certainty. Another major limitation of the QALY approach is that it views quality of life from a very narrow perspective. Pain, distress and reduced mobility are the only factors taken into account. Although health is a significant influence on the quality of an individual's life, other factors also play an important role in determining quality. Human relationships and friendship, security, economic status, culture and society all have an effect on the quality of life. Moreover, individual perceptions vary as to what factors affect the quality of lives. For example, the effects of reduced mobility may be exacerbated, if an individual lives on the tenth floor of a high rise block of flats, where the lifts are constantly out of action making it impossible to leave the home. The same degree of immobility might be acceptable to an individual living in a bungalow adapted to accommodate a wheel chair, which makes it relatively simple to leave and enter home. However, presumably Williams is interested in those aspects of quality of life that can be directly affected by health care. QALYs are a tool of health care allocation and their scope is, therefore, limited.

The QALY implies that a rational person would trade additional years of life expectancy for an improved quality of life. Williams (1985) uses the example of a person undergoing coronary artery bypass graft surgery to support this claim and suggests that even though the individual's life expectancy might not change or might even be worse, they often still wish to undergo surgery in the hope that the reduction of the pain of severe angina will improve their quality of life. This seems plausible and there is, indeed, considerable potential for the QALY to be used as a tool to assist an individual to choose between different treatment options in order to decide which would bring the most benefit in terms of quality and quantity of life. However, in some circumstances, pain and immobility may be preferable to a more immediate death. An individual may be prepared to suffer considerable pain and distress in order to achieve future life-goals. In fact, goals are paramount when deciding what counts as a benefit. Even short-term goals, such as the opportunity to see family and friends or spend one more Christmas together, can be significant and factors other than quality of life may sometimes be relevant when deciding what counts as a benefit. However, it is also important that an individual's goals are realistic and achievable and the costs to society not so great that others suffer.

Individual choice is important, but the individual's desire to go on living is not the only consideration when deciding who to treat from a group of patients competing for the same scarce resource. I might be able to judge the worth of my own life, but I cannot compare it to the life of another and claim that my life is more valuable. Limited resources create competition and individual choices have to be reconciled and weighed against the competing claims of others.

Case Study

June is 35 years of age and a single parent with a daughter aged four years. She was diagnosed as having cancer of the breast three years ago and a recent CT Scan has confirmed widespread metastases. The health care team discuss with June ways in which her pain and symptoms can be controlled, but do not advocate any further courses of chemotherapy or treatment. June becomes very distressed and explains that she wants to spend one last Christmas with her daughter and is prepared to suffer any amount of pain in order to achieve this goal. She has undertaken some research via the internet and has information about a new 'experimental' drug, which although very expensive and not widely available in this country has had good results in a recent trial in the United States of America.

The health care team discuss her request and take the view that this treatment might bring some, but only very limited benefit in terms of increased life expectancy. However, to achieve her goal, June only requires months in terms of increased life expectancy not years. The effectiveness of the treatment is uncertain and the cost would be considerable and therefore prohibitive. In addition, if the drug was made available to June, to maintain fairness and equality it would also have to be made available to anyone else with a similar need. The high cost of this treatment for a few patients would mean sacrificing the extensive counselling and support service the authority were able to offer a large number of patients diagnosed with cancer. The team felt that this resulted in greater aggregate benefit, although perhaps at the expense of the individual.

- Does June have a justified claim to limited health care resources?
- Should we always seek to maximise the aggregate benefit of health care?
- In relation to your own area of clinical practice what treatments would you include and what treatments would you exclude?

Micro-allocation

The final selection of patients for treatment remains the most controversial. Selection of individuals competing for the same scarce resource cannot be made solely on the basis of medical considerations. Health care need, the capacity to benefit from treatment, and quality of life, have all been used in the selection of patients, but all are value laden concepts which are difficult to define and quantify. Impersonal mechanisms, such as lotteries and waiting lists, have also been advocated as well as biological age. But, in times of scarcity, a choice has to be made as to who to treat and this can sometimes mean hard choices regarding 'who shall live when not everyone can live,' (Beauchamp and Childress, 1994: 365). Is there a fair, rational and morally defensible way to decide who should receive the resource and if so, what selection criteria should be used?

Random selection: first come, first served

Selecting individuals for treatment on a first come, first served basis is a form of random selection traditionally used in medicine to decide which individual to treat first if resources are inadequate, or in order to decide the priority in which patients are admitted to hospital or treated in an A&E department. It functions as a sort of 'natural lottery' and shares similarities with a lottery which is the other main form of random selection (Kilner, 1990: 194). This approach is rarely used as a primary method of allocation, but as a means of making a final choice once other criteria, such as medical need, have been met.

A first come, first served approach does have advantages. Individuals usually become ill at random intervals, therefore, as they become ill they are considered for whatever resources they need. If the resources are unavailable, the individual would have either to wait or go elsewhere, but if they wait would be assured of treatment before anyone arriving after them. It would usually be possible to give some indication of how long the wait would be and this approach would ensure that eventually each individual had a chance of receiving the resource, providing of course they did not die while waiting for the resource to become available. This method of selection is easy to apply and less costly to administer in terms of financial and human costs than other selection methods. It does not require information about candidates to be collected and assessed, which is a costly process, often inaccurate, might involve the formation of selection committees, and is also time-consuming and therefore impractical in situations where, without the swift instigation of life-sustaining treatment, the individual might die. Moreover, it is suggested that the first come, first served method is less costly psychologically as it saves the decision-makers the anguish and guilt of having to compare lives in order to save some and leave others to die (Broome, 1984: 39).

However, it would still be possible for prejudice and bias to enter even a first come, first served selection method. The individual has to be given the opportunity of a chance of waiting. Other criteria would have to be utilised to decide which candidates warranted treatment in the first place and were granted the opportunity of waiting. This decision is usually based on medical need. A health care professional may delay seeing a patient or refuse to put his/her name on the waiting list. Even a few minutes' delay could make a vital difference to the outcome for an individual requiring life-sustaining treatment. Alternatively, the individual who had waited the longest would be treated first, which could be at the expense of treating the individual with the greatest health care need. Although a first come, first served method of random selection might ensure each individual had an equal chance of receiving the resource, this might only have been achieved at the expense of treating the candidate who is more likely to benefit from treatment. Important factors such as survivability would not be taken into account.

Case Study

An individual with a very limited chance of survival arrives at a district general hospital and is admitted to the last bed on the intensive care unit. Shortly afterwards, another individual arrives who also requires this facility. In this instance, the individual has a potentially recoverable condition and a much better chance of survival with full recovery.

- Should priority still be given to the individual who arrived first whose prognosis is poor or to the individual with a greater likelihood of benefit?

Beauchamp and Childress (1994: 383) argue that admission to an intensive care unit does not give an individual an absolute claim for priority treatment, and that it would sometimes be morally justified to discharge someone to make room for another with a greater medical need and prospect of success. But, in this instance, a decision to initiate treatment has already been made and treatment begun. An individual's condition or response to treatment may well change, rendering care on such a unit inappropriate; but the decision to withdraw treatment should be made for this reason and independently of whether another individual is waiting to receive the resource. This practice is incompatible with the health care professionals duty of care towards the patient and would place intolerable burdens upon both the individual and his/her family as they would feel a constant sense of insecurity as treatment might be discontinued at any moment. Therefore, prioritising and treating individuals on a first come, first served basis might mean than an individual with a greater likelihood of benefit is sacrificed.

The capacity to benefit is considered to be an important consideration to avoid resources being wasted and ensure efficiency and effectiveness. However, as previously stated, equality is also an important principle and selecting patients on a first come, first served approach does ensure that each individual has an equal chance of receiving the resource, although only one candidate is actually chosen. But, when efficiency and equity conflict, does one weigh each competing principle against another?

Medical need

It is often assumed that medical resources should be distributed according to the degree of health care need, as this
method of selection takes into account the needs of the individual without reference to or comparison with others
(Kilner, 1990: 115). Selection of individuals for treatment
on this basis does initially appear simple, straightforward
and rational. There is little point in giving treatment to
someone who does not need it; to do so would be wasteful
and inefficient and could subject patients to considerable
physical and psychological harm. Need must be an important consideration, but, in times of scarcity when resources
are limited, problems arise deciding who should be selected
for treatment from a group of candidates with similar, but
competing medical need. Other non-medical criteria might
need to be considered, such as the capacity to benefit from
treatment. So, questions arise, concerning the following:

- Defining and quantifying need
- Deciding which patient has the greatest need if several patients are competing for the same scarce
  resource with similar but different types of need
- Making a judgment about whether an individual will
  actually benefit from treatment
- Deciding where despite a health care need treatment
  is needed, wanted or necessary.

A health care need can be either instrumental (needed for a
purpose) or non-instrumental, or categorical (essential for
survival) (Wiggins, 1987). The distinction is not always
clear or well-defined. For example, there are health care
needs associated with enhancing quality of life (the need for
effective relief from the constant pain of arthritis). There
are also needs associated with survival (the need for renal
dialysis or life-sustaining treatment on an intensive care
unit). Alternatively, people sometimes need things to prevent other needs arising (including preventive primary
health care, such as health education and vaccination
programmes). Harris (1996) argues that life-sustaining

treatment should always take priority as not to do so would result in the sacrifice of the life of one person who is very ill and expensive to treat, in order to make a tiny improvement to the aggregate health status of the community. But preventive care is sometimes more effective and efficient than critical care in saving lives, and it does not automatically follow that life-sustaining treatment should always take precedence over life-enhancing or preventive care. Allocating resources only to treat present dangers would ruin preventive health care and jeopardise future lives (Culyer, 1997). Health needs are limitless, and whether a need is defined as instrumental or non-instrumental often depends on who assesses or categorises the need. One health care professional might equate a categorical need with pain and distress, while another might refer to how imminent death is (New and Grand, 1996: 56). Hence, making the distinction between a non-instrumental and instrumental sense of health care need is problematic and open to individual interpretation.

A health care need does not necessarily mean that treatment is needed or is necessary. An individual may have a health care need, but not need treatment, perhaps because there is no effective treatment available to meet the need. For example, an individual with terminal cancer may have a need, but the treatment available has proved to be ineffective in meeting this need (a return to health). Further invasive treatment might be deemed unnecessary (although there would still be a need for effective palliative care). There is often more than one way of meeting a patient's need and, although there might not be a need for treatment, there might be a need to provide more effective palliative care or undertake further research in order to provide more effective treatment (Culyer, 1995). An individual may have a medical need that could be met by initiating treatment; for example, renal dialysis to maintain renal function. However, this does not mean that treatment should be initiated. Other additional economic and ethical factors need to be considered, such as whether the patient wants treatment and the capacity to benefit from treatment in terms of quality as well as number of life-years gained.

Selection of individuals for treatment on the basis of need does not necessarily mean the equitable, effective or efficient use of scare resources. The likelihood of the patient benefiting from treatment also has to be considered to avoid resources being wasted. Indeed, Culyer (1995) argues that, if an individual cannot benefit from treatment, they do not need it. But, how ill the patient is, is not the same question as how much the patient can benefit from treatment. This is a function of what the treatment can do and how effective the treatment is, not how ill the patient is. Although these additional considerations may affect the decision-making process, it is important that the reason treatment is not initiated is explicitly stated and made clear as, all too often, the reason is given as 'the patient does not need treatment'. This does not reflect an honest assessment of need and avoids health care professionals' explicitly denying individuals resources. This practice can be potentially harmful as it prevents individuals from seeking treatment or help from other available sources (Kilner, 1990:117).

The use of health care need as a criterion for selecting candidates competing for the same scarce resource has considerable limitations and, even if a workable concept of need could be adopted, an individual's health care need alone fails to provide justification and is not a sufficient basis for allocating scarce resources. Selecting patients for treatment on the sole basis of need can conflict with, and be at the expense of, treating those patients who are more likely to benefit from treatment. This can lead to unacceptable outcomes and result in huge amounts of resources being devoted to individuals with no capacity or significant chance to benefit from treatment (New and Grand, 1996: 57). Other non-medical criteria also needs to be considered, such as the patient's age and quality of life, which affect the capacity to benefit from treatment.

Capacity to benefit from treatment

Benefit is the most widely used and advocated criterion in the UK to make decisions regarding treatment options. Benefit is measured in terms of length of years of gained, quality of life and the success or efficiency of treatment. Cost-benefits are also a consideration (Harris, 1996). The justification for this approach is that it is wasteful to give someone with a very small chance of survival the same priority for treatment as someone with a much better chance, even if they have the same medical need. In order to maximise the expected outcome or benefit of treatment, the patient with a 90% chance of survival would always be preferred and chosen for treatment as opposed to the patient with only a 50% chance. This method of prioritisation could result in patients with equal need or those more in need of urgent life-saving treatment being denied care in favour of those in whom treatment is deemed more likely to succeed. There is a need to protect against waste, but what counts as a benefit and how benefit is measured requires careful consideration. Any measure of benefit or outcome needs to take a broad range of medical, ethical and economic factors into account, including:

- Should only health benefits be taken into account. What about other non-related benefits?
- Does an individual's claim on health care resources rest on the size of the benefit gained—bigger being better?
- How is a choice made if the size of the benefit to be gained from treatment is roughly equal amongst competing candidates?

Quality of life

Decisions to withhold or withdraw health care treatment have always been influenced by judgments regarding the capacity of the patient to benefit from treatment in terms of quality of life as well as the length of additional years gained. Both are important considerations when deciding who should receive treatment. However, quality of life is a broad concept, encompassing many different aspects of an individual's life and ability to function and enjoy life. It is, therefore, a difficult concept to define and quantify. To make a judgment which involved comparing and measuring the quality of different patients' lives would require the health care professional to be clear about the concept being measured. The QALY is a useful tool to help individuals to choose and compare the benefits of different treatment options. However, the use of QALYs at a micro-level of resource allocation to choose between competing candidates might result in choosing the candidate without pre-existing disease or disability, or those with diseases that are less expensive to treat. The QALY would also favour treating the candidate with the probability of greater life expectancy. This is not necessarily unfair or discriminatory, for in times of scarcity, the capacity to benefit from treatment has to be considered; but, as previously discussed, what counts as a benefit and how this is measured requires careful consideration, and factors other than quality of life may need to be taken into account. In its present form, the QALY approach fails to provide an adequate measure as it views benefit from a very narrow and limited perspective.

Age

The use of biological age has been advocated as a criterion for rationing limited resources (Clarke, 2001). Although an explicit policy of rationing by age within the UK has not been formulated, decisions to withhold or withdraw treatment are already being made on the basis of the patient's biological age rather than medical need (Shaw, 1994). The use of age as a selection criterion is, therefore, implicit and often disguised as a form of medical benefit criterion (Kilner, 1990: 82). The use of age as a selection criterion has considerable appeal as it is objective and precise. However, denying individuals treatment and the use of new technologies solely on the basis of their age is viewed by some as unfair and discriminatory, with the potential to cause conflict between generations (Rivlin, 1995).

Nursing issues

Health care professionals are an expensive and sometimes scarce human resource, who constantly have to make decisions about how to prioritise care when individuals compete for their time and attention. This may not be a life and death decision, but it is nonetheless problematic. In addition, nurses develop a relationship and have a duty of care towards each individual patient, and this can create difficulties and conflict when attempting to balance the needs of the individual against the needs of society as a whole. The knowledge that limited resources has meant a hard choice between competing individuals and the delivery of less than optimal care can also generate feelings of distress and discomfort.

An exercise

Consider a situation that might arise in your own area of clinical practice, where you have had to make a difficult choice between individual patients with a similar health care need who are competing for your time and attention.

- What considerations might be relevant to the choice and why?

References

Beauchamp TL, Childress JF (1994) *Principles of Biomedical Ethics*. 4th edn. Oxford University Press, USA

Broome J (1984) Selecting people randomly. *Ethics* **95**: 38–55

Clarke CM (2001) Rationing scarce life-sustaining resources on the basis of age. *J Adv Nurs* **35**(5): 799–804

Culyer AJ (1997) The rationing debate: Maximising the health of the whole community: The case for. *Br Med J* **314**(7081): 667–69

Culyer AJ (1995) Need: The idea won't do—but we still need it. *Soc Sci Med* **40**(6): 727–30

Fried C (1983) An analysis of 'equality' and 'rights' in medical care. In: Arras J, Hunt R, eds. *Ethical Issues in Modern Medicine*. Mayfield Publishing, Maidenhead

Harris J (1996) What is the good of health care? *Bioethics* **10**(4): 269–91

Hunter DJ (1997) *Desperately Seeking solutions: Rationing Health Care*. Longman. London

Kilner JF (1990) *Who Lives? Who Dies? Ethical Criteria in Patient Selection*. Yale University Press, New Haven, USA

Mostafa SM (1995) The cost of an intensive care unit. *Care Critically Ill* **11**(1): 28–31

New B, Grand JL (1996) *Rationing in the NHS*. Kings Fund, London

Rivlin MM (1995) Protecting elderly people: flaws in ageist arguments. *Br Med J* **310**: 1179–82

Shaw B (1994) In defence of ageism. *J Med Ethics* **20**: 188–91

Singer P (1994) *Rethinking Life and Death. The Collapse of Our Traditional Ethics*. Oxford University Press, Oxford

Wiggins D (1987) Needs, need, needing. *J Med Ethics* **13**: 62–68

Williams A (2001) Dilemmas in health care: responding to economic constraints. In: Konaromy C, ed. *Dilemmas in UK Health Care*. The Open University, Buckingham

Williams A (1985) Economics of coronary artery bypass grafting. *Br Med J* **291**: 326–29

10

HEALTH CARE POLICY

P Warwick

Introduction

Box 10.1 What would you do?

As a recently appointed nurse in the Day Surgery Unit, one of the clerical staff explains to you that all your new colleagues advise vasectomy patients of one of the surgeons to have a general rather than local anaesthetic. This concerns you because you know that local anaesthetics are safer, usually take less time and cost less. When you ask why, you are told that the surgeon is in the habit of proceeding with operations before the local anaesthetic has fully taken effect; this has shown up on pain score surveys in multidisciplinary audit meetings but nothing happened as a result.

- Should you do something about it? Is there anything you can do? How might Clinical Governance impact on this?

Successful and effective professionals understand the environment in which they operate. This chapter attempts to explain the wider organisational and political environment by focussing on health policy and management issues, which relate to the ethical agenda covered elsewhere in the book. Some ethical dilemmas may occur at a very personal level involving one individual patient; however, a far greater number arise as a result of the apparently conflicting demands of individual health need and the management of health care resources. An understanding of health policy is thus an important step in professional and personal development.

In this chapter, ethics has been interpreted in its widest possible sense, including morals, codes of conduct and values as well as more obvious ethical issues. Values are particularly relevant to health policy because the values held by the government have a big impact on the organisation of health care. To what extent the government reflects the views of society and to what extent it shapes those views is a question for another book, but, for our purposes, I think we have to accept there is a close link.

In the UK, there has long been tension between public and private sector provision of public services (Martin and Henderson, 2001). On one side of the argument, there is the concern for the size of the tax bill and an argument that a greater proportion of public sector funding should be paid for privately and, on the other side, the view that there should be universally available, dependable public services. Early in the twenty-first century, it appears that the latter argument is winning the day and that the values of society demand a modern and dependable health service for all (Department of Health, 1997); this view is reflected in government health policy, as we shall see. One consequence of societal demands for modern health care is the increasing expectations of patients and their carers. The Government repeatedly tells the electorate that more money is being put into health care and as a result we expect that we will get better services. Increased expectations mean more choices between competing demands and more decisions to be made about what is and what is not going to be provided. Is this rationing of health care? We will look at how this implicit rationing of health care is managed.

Health care policy in the UK has always been based on the medical model, with the health professional, particularly the doctor, as the central figure around whom services are organised. Changing public values are challenging this situation, so that the NHS of the early twenty-first century is more likely to have the patient or client as the central figure around whom services are planned and provided. In this chapter, we will try to look at the main drivers of these developments. We will look at quality improvement and other developments that go under the banner of Modernisation.

In recent years, there have been a number of appalling incidents of unethical and criminal behaviour by health care professionals. The recent list of names and incidents includes Allitt, Shipman, The Royal Liverpool Children's Hospital, The Victoria Climbie Inquiry and the Bristol heart surgeons. One response to these incidents has been to increase the legislation and controls imposed on professions that had previously been largely left to self-regulate. We look at the policy and legislation in this area, in particular the role of Clinical Governance and the new regulating bodies.

One potential consequence of recent developments in health care policy in the UK is that a more regulated, risk-averse service is less likely to push out the boundary of medical care and make a breakthrough in a new type of treatment. We will look at the regulatory framework for health care research, in particular the role of the ethical committee and touch on the role of the Human Genetics Commission.

Finally, we will look at the expectation that public servants behave with honesty and integrity. In the autumn of 2002, a new Code of Conduct was introduced for managers of health care; the values are similar to those introduced by the Nolan Committee's First Report on Standards in Public Life (www.official-documents.co.uk). We will look at the code and consider implications for health care professionals working at all levels in the NHS.

In summary, the purpose of the chapter is to:

- Identify and explain the main policy documents and circulars that form a backdrop to ethical decision-making and discussions about the quality of patient care
- Analyse the ethical issues that arise when attempting to manage health

- Using case studies, apply some of the ideas and concepts to the sort of health care settings in which recently qualified practitioners may find themselves working.

The framework

In 1997, a new Labour Government was elected, determined to reform and improve the public services. Next to education, health was the biggest focus of the 1997 general election campaign. Within a few months of the election, they had produced their new strategy for the NHS (Department of Health, 1997). This document not only reformed the internal market structure, and introduced Primary Care Groups and Primary Care Trusts, but also introduced the quality framework that has since become central to the way all health professionals function in the NHS. It introduced the concepts of national standards and frameworks, as set out in National Service Frameworks (NSFs) and the National Institute of Clinical Excellence (NICE), and a regulatory framework based on self-regulation, to be called Clinical Governance. A national body, The Commission for Health Improvement (CHI), was set up to oversee, inspect and tackle shortcomings in health care provision.

The detail of the new quality framework was put together in a quality strategy document, A First Class Service (Department of Health, 1998). This document contained the often-used diagram in *Figure 10.1*. This is variously known as the three-tier quality strategy, the clinical governance sandwich or the flying donuts diagram.

At the top of the diagram are the nationally agreed service standards, set out in the NSFs and by NICE. There are NSFs for Mental Health, Cancer Services, Coronary Heart Disease (CHD), Diabetes, Renal Services, Older People and a Children's Services Framework. NICE is the body charged with determining what treatments and technologies should be provided by the NHS. Occasionally, their decisions have hit the headlines, for example, the appraisal of beta interferon for the treatment of multiple sclerosis

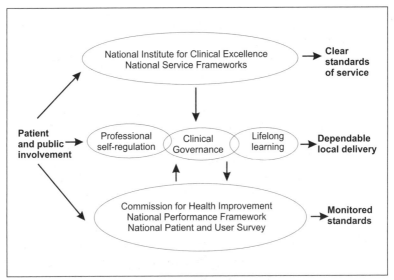

Figure 10.1: Setting, delivering and monitoring standards (A First Class Service, Department of Health, 1998)

(October 2001) and Relenza as a treatment for influenza in November 2000 (NICE News Archive, www.nice.org.uk). The overall objective of the Institute is to promote high clinical standards in the NHS by developing or commissioning guidance on clinical and cost-effectiveness, and disseminating this guidance to clinicians, patients and commissioners (NICE Board Meetings, www.nice.org.uk 2002).

The most noted aspect of NICE's role is the decisions it makes to provide or not provide treatment available to the public via the NHS. NICE takes advice from professionals and a Citizen's Council and has a Board made up of lay people, professionals, and managers. Decisions are not made on the basis of an ethical debate, but tend to be based on technical and economic considerations; however, inevitably decisions will be influenced by the values of those involved in the decision-making process, so that decisions are made based on implicit, even subconscious, ethical considerations rather than an explicit debate about the pros and cons of each decision made. To their credit, NICE do seemed to have embraced the concept of public involvement in the decision-making process, arguably more so than other health care organisations.

Rationing of services can be explicit, as in the case when health authorities in the past have been prepared to draw up clear criteria for the funding of cosmetic plastic surgery or invitro fertilisation (IVF) treatment. NICE also works in this way, by drawing up criteria and exclusions. However, other forms of rationing do take place on a more implicit basis; for instance, through barriers to services, such as the cost of dental care, waiting lists or the need to talk to a health professional before the provision of 'the morning after pill'

At the foot of the diagram in *Figure 10.1* is the monitoring or quality assurance part of the framework. Primary Care Trusts, Trusts and Strategic Health Authorities are required to submit performance assessment framework data, which are used for star rating purposes and made available for public scrutiny on the Department of Health website, (www.doh.gov.uk). The Commission for Health Improvement (CHI) has a rolling programme of Trust visits to ensure that they have adequate Clinical Governance arrangements in place. It also investigates specific allegations and care delivery problems in under-performing Trusts; for instance, one of the first of these investigations followed adverse publicity and poor standards of patient care in the North Lakeland Healthcare NHS Trust in November 2000: www.chi.nhs.uk). In 2004, CHI becomes the Commission for Health Audit and Inspection (CHAI) with a broader role, which includes the publication of performance rating 'league tables' and star status.

The third quality assurance element is the National Patient Survey. Surveys of GP patients, those suffering from CHD, cancer service patients and acute hospital inpatients have all been surveyed in this way. The scale and coverage of the latter survey will act as a useful yardstick in years to come, when similar surveys should reveal whether patients perceive improvements have been made.

In between national standards and the national quality assurance system is the local delivery level. This consists of strengthened professional self-regulation in the light of perceived failings with the old systems, strengthened requirements for continuous professional development, and, in the centre, the requirement for each NHS organisation to regulate its own clinical practice through Clinical Governance. A First Class Service defined Clinical Governance as:

> *'A Framework through which NHS organisations are accountable for continuously improving the quality of their services and safeguarding high standards of care by creating an environment in which excellence in clinical care will flourish.'*

(Department of Health, 1998: 33)

The Health Circular, HSC 1999/065, went on to detail how NHS organisations were supposed to implement Clinical Governance. The aim is to set up a framework and processes that enable staff to deliver quality services; with the processes in place, the hope is that incremental or step improvements in the service will continue to drive up the standard of services provided. A Clinical Governance framework should identify and build on good practice, assess and minimise the risk of untoward events, investigate problems and ensure lessons are learnt, and support health professionals to deliver quality care (Department of Health, 1998: 35). Disregard for the patient, sometimes an unfortunate consequence of the medical model of health care, is no longer acceptable and the values that condoned this type of approach no longer have a place in this new system.

Clinical governance arrangements also mean that chief executives are responsible for the clinical performance of their organisations and that board meetings should receive reports on clinical performance of the Trust, as well as financial and activity information. These reporting arrangements should, in theory, prevent the type of problem identified in *Box 10.1*. Previously, medical audit meetings might have reviewed a post-operative pain audit, but would have relied on individual practitioners to alter their practice. Unfortunately, this did not always happen; bad practice sometimes continued because there was no mechanism for ensuring that the corrective action discussed at meetings was put into place. Now, medical directors have to put Clinical Governance reports to Trust Board meetings (including the results of clinical audits) and chief executives are accountable for the clinical governance arrangements in their Trusts, so there are people accountable for ensuring that problems like the high pain scores identified in box 10.1 are considered, causes identified and corrective action taken. If these arrangements are not in place, then CHAI reviews should identify problems with clinical governance arrangements in Trusts (Clinical Governance reports on individual Trusts are available on the CHAI website: www.chai.nhs.uk). If all else fails, all health care organisations should have arrangements for raising concerns, sometimes referred to as 'whistle blowing'.

Apart from Clinical Governance, the other main drive to improve the quality of patient and client services in the NHS is termed 'modernisation'. This is not really in the scope of this book or chapter, but readers may have come across schemes to modernise services such as outpatient departments, accident and emergency services, and primary care premises. Linking all these schemes are the similar aims of reshaping services to make patient care and the customer the central focus of service provision, moving away from the medical model, which has tended to dominated the design of NHS services up to now. The Modernisation Agency has become a significant force in the NHS, helping organisations to improve patient/client services. See the Modernisation Agency website: http:///www.modernnhs.nhs.uk for further details.

In Spring 2003, a new NHS Quality Strategy was published. Called, 'Raising Standards—Improving Performance in the NHS, the emphasis in this new strategy is targeting funding at Trusts which have been rated as no star or one star by CHAI. The aim being to have all Trusts graded as three star, by 2008.

Learning lessons

The NHS has had many scandals since its inception, but arguably few have had as much lasting impact as those that unfolded in the 1990s and early in the 2000s. Beverly Allitt, a paediatric nurse, was convicted of killing four children and seriously injuring several more. Harold Shipman, a single-handed GP working in Greater Manchester, was convicted of killing 15 patients (www.news.bbc.uk, 31 January 2000) and suspected of having many more victims over his career. In Bristol, complicated heart surgery on sick children continued despite consistently bad results over ten or more years. The Inquiry calculated that between 30 and 35 deaths occurred as a result of a combination of poor clinical practice and poor management arrangements at the Bristol Royal Infirmary (Bristol Royal Infirmary Inquiry 2001 also known as The Kennedy Report). These three incidents in particular had a significant impact on the public's perception of the caring professions. The Government needed to be seen to be changing the values of the organisation and in response several significant circulars and new arrange- ments have been put in place.

In 2000, the Chief Medical Officer (CMO) attempted to set about changing the values and culture of the professionally-dominated organisation in his report on learning from adverse incidents—An Organisation with a Memory (Department of Health, 2000). This circular called for a new culture in which health care professionals could learn from adverse events and near misses, in a similar way to the aviation industry, rather than failing to report incidents in a climate of fear and punishment. The circular proposed the creation of the National Patients Safety Agency and a national reporting system for adverse incidents. The NHS Plan (Department of Health, 2000) declared the Government's commitment to implementing An Organisation with a Memory and the new agency was introduced in another circular, Building a Safer NHS for Patients (Department of Health, 2001).

The Government's response to the Bristol Royal Infirmary Inquiry, Learning from Bristol (Department of Health,

2002), catalogues all the patient safety, professional regulation and quality improvement arrangements that the current government has put in place since its election to office in 1997. This is an interesting read and a useful report to help understand the jargon and the acronyms for all the new agencies and frameworks set up during this period. There is no specific mention of ethics, but much talk of values, culture and putting patients at the centre of the NHS. The report concludes that 'Bristol was a turning point in the history of the NHS' (*Summary: p5*) and that good will come out of the tragedy.

Research And Ethics Committees

Anyone conducting research in the area of health and social care should get prior approval of this research from their research ethics committee (REC). These previously operated differently in each trust and health authority but new guidance was presented in the Research Governance Framework, published in September 2002, which set out the broad principles for the governance of research and a national framework of committees to adjudicate on the ethics of research proposals. All research proposals involving one or more of the following must be referred to an REC:

- NHS patients and service users
- Relatives and carers of patients or users
- Organs or bodily material of current or former patients
- Foetal material
- Recently deceased patients
- NHS premises or facilities
- NHS staff working in their NHS jobs

(Department of Health, 2002)

The role of RECs is to provide independent advice to researchers on the ethics of research proposals, their primary purpose being to protect the dignity, rights, safety and well-being of actual and potential participants. The new framework introduces standardised procedures across the NHS for managing research proposals, and introduces a set of standardised REC forms. A national body, the Central Office for Research Ethics Committees (COREC) coordinates the work of RECs, manages research proposals that cover more than one REC, and acts as an information and training resource for people involved in RECs. Further regulations apply to work involving prisoners, gene therapy, human fertilisation and embryology, and animal to human transplant activity (xenotransplantation). Details can be found on the Human Genetics Commission website, www.hgc.gov.uk.

Management ethics

Box 10.2: What would you do?

Almost one in ten health managers say that they have fiddled figures to make it look like their organisation is meeting government targets (BBC News Health 10/11/02). Staff said they were under pressure from Government officials and Civil Servants at NHS Executive Regional Offices to record the required figures and that they were afraid to raise any concerns. Patient activity figures were, therefore, subject to manipulation to ensure that they gave the required rather than the correct picture.

It is apparent from this news report that that the very Ministers and Trust Managers who are charged with ensuring that doctors, nurses and other health professionals work in a moral and ethical way, find it impossible themselves to adhere to such standards and find it almost impossible to raise concerns because of a climate of fear and perceived threat.

- How would you react if you become a service manager in this situation? Would you tow the line or speak out and risk intimidation, harassment or losing your job? Could regulations make a difference?

Criticism of health care professionals, such as the Bristol heart surgeons, has prompted government action to tighten up the regulation of nurses, medical and allied health professionals; similarly, criticism of NHS managers (among other things for manipulating waiting list figures, see *Box 10.2*) led to the development of a Code of Conduct for NHS Managers. The Code, published in October 2002, says that it has two purposes: to guide NHS managers in the work that they do and choices that they make and to reassure the public. The code states that it applies to all managers (presumably from supervisors and E grade nurses in charge of shifts upwards) and is to be written into their terms and conditions of service, even those of the most senior managers in NHS organisations. *Figure 10.2* contains the main principles of the Code:

As an NHS manager, I will observe the following principles:

- make the care and safety of patients my first concern and act to protect them from risk;

- respect the public, patients, relatives, carers, NHS staff and partners in other agencies;

- be honest and act with integrity;

- accept responsibility for my own work and the proper performance of the people I manage;

- show my commitment to working as a team member by working with all my colleagues in the NHS and the wider community;

- take responsibility for my own learning and development.

Figure 10.2: Code of Conduct for NHS Managers

You might like to consider the impact of this document on the survey reported in *Box 10.2*. Will the code lead to a change of practice? Will senior managers in the NHS become more ethical because they have a Code of Conduct or will they still make people working for them feel under pressure and afraid to raise concerns?

The second paragraph of the Code of Conduct states: 'I will respect and treat with dignity and fairness, the public, patients relatives, carers, NHS staff and partners in other agencies.' This a fine aspiration which attracts almost universal support among managers who would like to think that they do indeed respect the public, patients and staff, but it seems to have little influence on the actions of some senior managers when a member of the public objects to the reorganisation of acute hospital services, when a patient is patronised with jargon in response to a complaint or when an intimidated member of staff is expected to work long hours that compromises his or her work/life balance. Breaches of the Code are investigated internally or externally if the chief executive or directors are under investigation. The outcome of investigations will determine the impact of the Code. There does seem to be the potential for numerous complaints about breaches of the Code by unscrupulous managers; however, in the two years following its publication, no challenges were reported in the public arena.

One of the problems faced by health managers is that they have an almost impossible job, balancing the competing demands for resources, trying to hit unrealistic, imposed deadlines, trying to ensure staff are empowered to be innovative, but kept in check at the same time, maintaining standards of care while dealing with every patient referred to their service. Is it fair? Is it ethical for the Government ministers to expect the service to be managed within a limited budget? Is it ethical for those same ministers to sack managers who fail to meet some of their targets? Given that the stakes are so high, is it surprising that managers are occasionally tempted to manipulate their performance returns?

Further complicating the manager's task, and often impacting on health care professionals doing their daily jobs, are party politics and the partisan politically motivated national and local press. It could be argued that health care professionals have to act in a way that is both ethical and politically wise. Ethics and politics can some times cause dilemmas for health practitioners, as in the case of Rose Addis in January 2002 (BBC News February 2002; see *Box 10.3* at the end of the chapter).

Nursing Issues: What Does This Mean For Me?

Nurses need to be aware of the organisational and policy environment in which they work, so that they can practice in a professional and ethical manner, act as effective advocates for their clients and patients, and know how to put a case for extra resources. They must also plan and manage their continuing professional development and have an understanding of organisational, as well as personal development needs.

This chapter, written by an ex-health service manager, has a managerial slant. It presents a range of information that should help newly qualified nurses to understand and know enough about the issues covered to contribute to staff meetings and ask pertinent questions of their managers. In particular, understanding the quality strategy illustrated in *Figure 10.1* will help them to understand the role of the various good practice guidelines, inspectors and auditors and will set clinical governance in context. Too often, the term 'clinical governance' is bandied about staff rooms and team meetings, without being defined or explained; one suspects that few really have a picture of what it is.

Depending on the area in which the newly qualified nurse works, NSFs, NICE rulings and public involvement may have differing roles and different degrees of impact; but, across the service, they are going to continue to be a significant influence for the duration of the current Government and quite possibly beyond. Students applying for jobs or newly qualified staff working in the areas covered by an NSF are particularly encouraged to read the NSF appropriate to their service.

The impact of An Organization with a Memory (Department of Health, 2000) should also be understood. The importance of reporting critical incidents, near misses and untoward incidents has to be set in the context of preventing further scandals and unnecessary patient suffering. Research by Vincent *et al* (2001) estimated that nearly 11% of all NHS patients suffer at least one adverse event during their care. A third of these incidents lead to a deterioration in the patient's condition and half of the incidents were avoidable with current standards of care. The estimated cost of the avoidable incidents was £1 billion (based on the cost of an average extra bed day). It is not surprising, given these figures, that the Government and the health professions are united in trying to cut down the number of adverse incidents and in setting up systems and a culture that allows NHS staff to analyse and learn from mistakes rather than conceal these events.

Any nurse or student undertaking research for a project or an academic assignment needs to be aware of the Research Governance Framework, which introduces a consistent policy and standards for research across the NHS. It is traditionally understood that any research involving patient data has to go through an Ethics Committee. This is also now the case for anyone doing research which, for instance, includes interviewing colleagues and members of staff or looking at NHS premises and equipment. It is too early to assess the impact of these guidelines, save to suggest that anyone planning any research on these lines needs to get to their local Research Ethics Committee early, as their agenda is likely to be a lot fuller than it has been in the past.

Finally, nurses do need to be aware that those in a managerial position are now subject to managerial codes of conduct as well as professional codes. For example, anyone not treating their staff with respect, or not allowing team members to strike an acceptable work/life balance are in breach of the Code of Conduct for NHS Managers and leave themselves open to challenge on this basis.

An exercise

The case of Rose Addis dominated the British press and was a leading television news item for over a week at the end of January and in early February 2002. It was debated in the Houses of Parliament and saw NHS staff and politicians exchanging insults. Let us consider the ethical issues in this case. What would you have done as a staff nurse in A&E involved in the initial treatment of this patient?

Following a fall at home, Rose Addis was taken to The Whittington Hospital Accident and Emergency Department in North London, at 11. 50 on the morning on 13th January 2002. Her daughter was contacted, rang to say she could not get to the hospital, but was assured that her mother was in a 'comfortable condition'. When her family did visit on 17th January they were not happy about her treatment and immediately raised their concerns with their MP, Iain Duncan Smith (who happened to be Leader of the Conservative opposition party) and the London Evening Standard. They alleged that Mrs Addis had been in A&E for 48 hours in the same clothes and had not been washed. They said they were told there were no beds for her in the hospital and that is why she was still in A&E.

Seeing an opportunity to attack his opposite number, Mr Duncan Smith almost immediately raised the case of Mrs Addis in the House of Commons at Prime Minister Question Time. The family's allegation, relayed by Mr Duncan Smith in Parliament, was that Mrs Addis had been treated 'worse than a dog', outraged hospital staff. The Trust's Medical Director appeared on the main evening news programmes the same evening, implying that Mrs Addis had been an awkward patient who had indicated that she did not want to be treated by some of the staff in the A&E department. He said she had remained under observation in A&E and that this was not unusual. The media interpreted this statement to the effect that she had not wanted to be treated by black members of staff—the Trust refused to confirm or deny this point.

Box 10.3: The Rose Addis Affair

At The Evening Standard, the story of a little old lady mistreated in an A&E Department was used to full effect. They said that it illustrated the state of the NHS in the capital city and revealed new aspects of the story for several days. The Chief Executive wrote a letter that stated that she had received prompt treatment, and that it would not be appropriate to wash her hair until her wound had healed. He said that she had been treated in an Accident and Emergency ward. She had refused to allow staff to undress her until her daughter arrived two days after admission and had continued to be most particular about whom she would allow to care for her.

For over a week at the end of January and early February 2002, claim and counter-claim were made by politicians, staff from the Hospital and the Evening Standard about Mrs Addis's treatment. The argument moved on to breaches of confidentiality, with all parties accusing each other of naming the patient and failing to maintain confidentiality. The political sympathies of the Trust's Medical Director also were made public knowledge in a bid to discredit his intervention (See BBC News 04/02/02)

Box 10.3: The Rose Addis Affair (contd)

Questions:

1. What should be the response of staff to overtly racist patients, who want to pick and chose the staff that treat them?

2. Should the views of 'difficult' or confused patients be ignored, if they are at odds with what might be best practice treatment?

3. Should an NHS Trust publicly defend its reputation and that of its staff in the light of aggressive accusations from aggrieved relatives, the media, or politicians, even if this means confirming the treatment of a member of the public?

4.   Staff were apparently unimpressed by the lack of concern shown by a family for their relative (it took two days for them to visit her), leading to suggestions that the complaint was a way of compensating for their absence. Should an apparent lack of sympathy shown by carers affect the way that they are informed about patient/client conditions?

Summary

In this chapter, we have looked at the wider context in which ethics are applied in health care settings. In particular, we have looked at the framework for clinical governance and quality management, and the impact of recent cases of unethical health care practices. Some of the scandals and bad practices have led to major changes in health policy, for example, the introduction of the National Patient Safety Agency. We have looked at the role of Ethics Committees and finished by debating some ethical considerations that relate to the management of health care.

Further Reading

Most of the references in this chapter relate to circulars, which are easily available on the Department of Health web site.

The New NHS modern, dependable is the 1997 NHS strategy document of the newly elected Labour Government. *A First Class Service* (1998) identified the quality strategy and introduced the two new bodies, CHI and NICE, as well as giving more detail about the concept of Clinical Governance. *The NHS Plan* (2000) updates the Government's health strategy and forms a statement of intent for major reforms and modernisation of the NHS.

The Bristol Royal Infirmary Inquiry Report (*The Kennedy Report*), *The Government's response*, *The Liverpool Children's Hospital Inquiry* and *An Organisation with a Memory* would be would be worth looking at if you want to

gain a better understanding of how management arrangements can break down to such an extent that unethical
practice went unchallenged for years and resulted in major
scandals when it was eventually exposed.

References

Bristol Royal Infirmary Inquiry, (2001) Final Report: www.bris-
tol-inquiry.org.uk/finalreport

The case that sparked a storm BBC News 23 January 2002:
www.news.bbc.uk

Martin V, Henderson E (2001) *Managing in Health and Social
Care*. Routledge, London

NHS managers fiddle figures, BBC News, 7 October 2002:
www.news.bbc.uk

NICE News Archive: www.nice.org.uk/ (accessed 14/11/02)

Nolan Committee's First Report on Standards in Public Life:
www.official-documnets.co.uk, (accessed 14/11/02)

The Royal Liverpool Children's Inquiry, (2001) Summary of
Report: www.rlcinquiry.org.uk/summary

Shipman jailed for 15 murders BBC News, 31 January 2000,
www.news.bbc.uk (accessed 27/2/2003)

Vincent C, Neal G, Woloshynowych M (2000) Adverse events in
British hospitals, preliminary retrospective record. Review
in: *Br Med J* **322**(3): 517–19

Circulars: (all available on www.dh.gov.uk)

Department of Health (2003) *Raising Standards—Improving
Performance in the NHS*. Department of Health, London

Department of Health (2002) *The Response to the Bristol
Inquiry Report*. Department of Health, London

Department of Health (2002) Research Governance Framework
for Health and Social Care: (www.doh.gov.uk/research/rd3/
nhsrandd/researchgovernance.htm)

Department of Health (2002) *Code of Conduct for NHS Managers*. Department of Health, London

Department of Health (2001) *Building a Safer NHS for
Patients*. Department of Health, London

Department of Health (2000) *An Organisation with a Memory*. Department of Health, London

Department of Health (2000) *The NHS Plan*. Department of Health, London

Department of Health (1998) *A First Class Service*. Department of Health, London

Department of Health (1997) *The New NHS, Modern Dependable*. NHS, London

HSC 1999/065 *Clinical Governance in the NHS*. Department of Health, London

Websites:

Commission for Health Audit and Inspection: www.chai.nhs.uk/

Commission for Health Improvement: www.chi.nhs.uk/

Human Genetics Commission: www.hgc.gov.uk/

National Institute For Clinical Excellence: www.nice.org/

NHS Modernisation Agency: www.modernnhs.nhs.uk/

Nolan Committee First Report: www.official-documents.co.uk/

Research Governance: www.doh.gov.uk/research

Index

Index